Core Concepts in Clinical Infectious Diseases (CCCID)

Core Concepts in Clinical Infectious Diseases (CCCID)

Carlos Franco-Paredes, MD, MPH
Division of Infectious Diseases,
Phoebe Putney Physician Group, Albany GA; and
Division of Infectious Diseases,
Hospital Infantil de México, Federico Gómez,
México City, México

AMSTERDAM • BOSTON • HEIDELBERG • LONDON
NEW YORK • OXFORD • PARIS • SAN DIEGO
SAN FRANCISCO • SINGAPORE • SYDNEY • TOKYO
Academic Press is an imprint of Elsevier

Academic Press is an imprint of Elsevier
125 London Wall, London EC2Y 5AS, UK
525 B Street, Suite 1800, San Diego, CA 92101-4495, USA
50 Hampshire Street, 5th Floor, Cambridge, MA 02139, USA
The Boulevard, Langford Lane, Kidlington, Oxford OX5 1GB, UK

British Library Cataloguing-in-Publication Data
A catalogue record for this book is available from the British Library

Library of Congress Cataloging-in-Publication Data
A catalog record for this book is available from the Library of Congress

ISBN: 978-0-12-804423-0

For information on all Academic Press publications
visit our website at http://store.elsevier.com/

Typeset by Thomson Digital

  Working together
to grow libraries in
developing countries

www.elsevier.com • www.bookaid.org

Publisher: Sara Tenney
Acquisition Editor: Linda Versteeg-buschman
Editorial Project Manager: Halima Williams
Production Project Manager: Julia Haynes
Designer: Matt Limbert

Dedication

**To Javi, Nico, Maribel, Lala, Maru, Manolo and Nona
To my patients and colleagues during my training
at Emory University, Atlanta GA**

"Pathogenicity is not the rule. Indeed, it occurs so infrequently and involves such a relatively small number of species, considering the huge population of bacteria on the earth, that it has a freakish aspect. Disease usually results from inconclusive negotiations for symbiosis, an overstepping of the line by one side or the other, a biologic misinterpretation of borders"

Thomas L. Germs. *N Engl. J Med* 1972; 287:553.

"So close no matter how far…"

Nothing Else Matters by Metallica

Contents

Preface

Any infection can lead to a life-threatening outcome depending on circumstances. Successful diagnosis and treatment of infectious processes requires an understanding of the predisposing conditions of the host, the mechanism of acquisition of the infection, and a consideration of the differential diagnostic approach in order to modify the natural history of the disease produced by the infectious pathogen.

Most textbooks about infectious diseases provide a comprehensive review of specific infectious agents and the diseases they produce in the human host. This book is not about acquiring the knowledge structure of infectious diseases that is usually presented in classic textbooks of infectious diseases. Instead, the approach of this book is about assisting health-care providers or students in refining the intellectual and creative process of putting the pieces together to achieve an accurate clinical diagnosis and establish effective interventions. This book is intended to bridge the gap between exhaustive academic textbooks and the realities and needs of routine clinical infectious diseases activities. The contents of this book are presented in an easy-to-use syndrome-based approach.

This book provides medical students, infectious disease fellows, and practicing clinicians with key clinical concepts in the differential diagnosis and workup of infectious diseases. With the use of tables and charts and through a syndrome-problem-oriented approach, it provides readers with a fresh approach of organizing knowledge and clinical experiences when caring for a fellow human being who is suffering from an infectious disease. Deeper knowledge improves patient care.

Chapter 1

Sepsis

DIAGNOSTIC APPROACH TO SEPSIS

We live in a world where nature rules. Man is irremediably embedded in nature with complex interactions with all living organisms. Ecologies vary across landscapes of built and natural environments, different geopolitical realities, and different access to health care and public health services.[1] Infectious pathogens do not rely on our anthropocentric spatial understanding for them to negotiate the negative spaces between human vision and the landscapes that afford them to reproduce and survive. This is true as it occurs in the dense jungle of the Amazonian river as well as in the modern setting of an intensive care unit in a highly specialized hospital.

In striving for self-transcendence and coexistence with other living organisms, our ancestors have experienced formidable molecular strife and have adopted ingenious adaptations.[2] As a result, with the progression from unicellular to multicellular life, bacteria have coexisted with humans. In this biological journey, we are shared, occupied, or rented with viruses, bacteria, archaea, protozoa and fungi.[3]

Although there are important benefits provided by bacterial guests to the human host living in complex relationships and becoming part of their microbiome, some bacteria are able to cause a wide spectrum of diseases. Yet, despite effective antimicrobial interventions and subsequent elimination of the inciting pathogen, many patients die as a consequence of the exuberant and inadequately regulated immune response to the infection.[4]

INFECTION

This is the process whereby an infectious pathogen adheres and invades normally sterile tissues. When the infectious process affects the parenchyma of an organ it may lead to *abscess* formation, whereas when an infectious pathogen invades existing spaces it may cause an *empyema*, for example, when a bacterial pathogen reaches the pleural space or the subdural space.

When viable bacteria reach the bloodstream and detected by blood cultures, this is defined as *bacteremia*. Similarly, when a viral pathogen is detected in peripheral blood through culture or by molecular detection assays, the patient is considered to have *viremia* (eg, CMV). When fungi, particularly some of the dimorphic fungi are detected in blood cultures, this is defined as *fungemia* (eg,

Core Concepts in Clinical Infectious Diseases (CCCID). http://dx.doi.org/10.1016/B978-0-12-804423-0.00001-9

TABLE 1.1 Infections Including Those Reaching the Bloodstream

Categories	Feature	Examples
Infection[a]	Adherence and invasion of sterile human tissues with clinical consequences[b,c]	Bacterial, viral, fungal, parasitic
Bacteremia	Detection of viable bacteria in the blood stream	Isolation of *Staphylococcus aureus* or *Streptococcus pneumonia* in a blood culture
Viremia	Detection of a virus or a viral component in the blood stream	Detection of cytomegalovirus (CMV) in transplant patients in a blood culture, antigenemia, or quantitative nucleic acid assays
Fungemia	Detection of fungal elements in the blood stream	Isolation of *Candida* or *Cryptococcus* in a blood culture
Parasitemia	Detection of a specific parasite in the bloodstream	Detection of *Trypanosoma cruzi* during the acute phase of Chagas disease in a peripheral blood smear; or detection of *Plasmodium falciparum* in a case of severe malaria in a peripheral blood smear

[a]*Infection of parenchyma often leads to abscess formation. Infection of existing spaces such as the pleural space of subdural spaces may result in an empyema.*
[b]*It is important to distinguish infection from disease since some microorganisms are consider colonizers of skin and mucosae but only in particular situations may become opportunistic pathogens (eg, oral candidiasis in an individual with AIDS). Disease-causing microbes include bacteria, virus, fungi, and parasites (protozoa and helminths).*
[c]*An important consideration relies on considering that infection leading to clinical manifestations (ie, disease) results often from the interaction between virulence factors of the infectious agent, the host response, and the need for environmental factors that allow transmission (the epidemiologic triangle). Sometime disease is produced by the ingestion or exposure to a pathogen toxin without evidence of replication in the human host.*

candidemia or cryptococcemia). Fungal blood cultures might rarely yield molds such as *Aspergillus* spp., particularly *Aspergillus terreus*, or *Fusarium* spp. *Parasitemia* may also be detected in peripheral blood in many protozoan infections such as in malaria, acute Chagas disease, babesiosis; or in helminthic infections (eg, filarial infections such as Loa loa) (Table 1.1).

SEPSIS

This is a clinical syndrome caused by an infection that stems from an uncontrolled or inadequately regulated inflammatory response with potential life-threatening consequences when it evolves into septic shock and multiorgan dysfunction syndrome (MODS).[5,6] The diagnostic criteria from sepsis include the presence of a confirmed or suspected source of infection associated with some of all of systemic inflammatory response syndrome (SIRS). In turn, a sequence of pathophysiologic events that may lead to end-organ damage, hemodynamic instability, and MODS may ensue after SIRS (Table 1.2). Sepsis occurs on a continuum of severity.

TABLE 1.2 Systemic Inflammatory Response Syndrome, Sepsis, Severe Sepsis, Septic Shock and Multiorgan Dysfunction Syndrome[a]

Condition	Distinguishing clinical features
Systemic inflammatory response syndrome (SIRS)[b]	Two or more of the following findings: • Fever (>38.3°C) or hypothermia (<36°C) • Tachycardia (heart rate > 90 beats/min or more than 2 SD above the upper limit of the normal range for age) • Leukocytosis (WBC > 12,000 cells/mm³), leukopenia (WBC < 4000 cells/mm³) or bandemia (>10%) • Tachypnea (respiratory rate > 20 breaths/min or a $PaCO_2$ < 32 mmHg indicating hyperventilation
Sepsis[c]	SIRS associated with a confirmed infectious process or when it is suspected
Severe sepsis[d]	Sepsis with end-organ damage/dysfunction including sudden onset of altered mental status, cardiac dysfunction, acute lung injury, lactic acidosis, decreased capillary refill time, mottled skin, ileus, hyperbilirrubinemia, hyperglycemia (in the absence of diabetes mellitus), thrombocytopenia or disseminated intravascular coagulopathy, decreased urine output, increased creatinine, or significant edema, and increased C-reactive protein or procalcitonin
Septic shock	Severe sepsis and systolic blood pressure less than 60 mmHg despite fluid challenge or requiring initiation of vasopressors to maintain systolic blood pressure above 60 mmHg
Refractory septic shock	Septic shock requiring higher dose of vasopressors (dopamine, norepinephrine, or epinephrine)
Multiorgan dysfunction syndrome	Dysfunction in one or more organs requiring interventions to maintain homeostasis

[a]The sequence of clinical progression may sometimes be inferred when under close observation of a patient in an ICU and may distinguish severe sepsis from septic shock. However, there is a continuum that it is often abrupt and indistinguishable clinically. Some individuals with septic shock or those with severe necrotizing pancreatitis and SIRS may progress rapidly to MODS and follow a fulminant course.
[b]SIRS may be caused by noninfectious causes such as pancreatitis, TTP, burns, trauma and others (see Table 1.3 and Figure 1.1 for pathogenesis based on exogenous versus endogenous factors).
[c]The 1991 American College of Chest Physicians/Society of Critical Care Medicine Consensus Conference established definition criteria. By 2001, the International Sepsis Definitions Conference broadened the classification to include hyperglycemia, increased C-reactive protein or procalcitonin, hyerplactatemia, decreased capillary refill, and hemodynamic instability or organ dysfunction.
[d]In 2003, a consensus panel endorsed the 1991/2001 definitions with the caveat that signs of a systemic inflammatory response, such as tachycardia or an elevated white blood cell count is not helpful in distinguishing sepsis from other conditions (infectious versus noninfectious). Thus, the term "severe sepsis" and "sepsis" are often used interchangeably to describe the syndrome of infection complicated by acute organ dysfunction (Angus DC, van der Poll T. Severe sepsis and septic shock. N Engl J Med 2013; 369(9): 840–851).

TABLE 1.3 Selected Clinical Syndromes Associated With Community-Acquired SIRS[a] or Sepsis

Condition	Etiology	Distinguishing clinical features
Meningococcemia	*Neisseria meningitidis* A/C/Y/W-135	Rapidly progressing sepsis Sometimes affecting those with terminal complement pathway deficiencies
Influenza	Influenza virus	Rhabdomyolysis Respiratory failure with bilateral interstitial infiltrates Rapidly progressing sepsis and multiorgan failure
Vibrio vulnificus	*V. vulnificus*	Affects mostly individuals with chronic liver disease or iron excess states. Recent exposure to seafood (oysters)
Acute endocarditis[b]	*S. aureus*	Associated with endovascular infection affecting endothelial cells of great vessels. Patients with persistent bacteremia
Acute bacterial meningitis	*S. pneumonia* *Haemophilus influenza* *N. meningitidis*	Patients with acute bacterial meningitis are frequently bacteremic
Necrotizing fasciitis/toxic shock syndrome	*Streptococcus pyogenes* *S. aureus*	Patients with *S. pyogenes* necrotizing fasciitis have often positive blood cultures in contrast with those with *S. aureus*
	Aeromonas hydrophila	Exposure to fresh water (estuary water)
Splenectomy[c]	Meningococcemia (*N. meningitides* A/C/Y/W-135)	Rapidly progressive sepsis
	Capnocytophaga canimorsus Babesiosis[d]	Dog-bite related
Tick-borne illnesses	Rocky Mountain spotted fever Ehrlichiosis Babesiosis	Febrile syndrome with headache, maculopapular rash, leukopenia, and elevated transaminases. Some patients progress rapidly to hemodynamic instability

TABLE 1.3 Selected Clinical Syndromes Associated With Community-Acquired SIRS[a] or Sepsis (*cont.*)

Condition	Etiology	Distinguishing clinical features
Melioidosis	*Burkholderia pseudomallei*	May occur in patients with diabetes mellitus or in patients with chronic granulomatous disease (other related pathogens that may present with sepsis in patients with phagocyte dysfunction include *Burkholderia gladioli*, *Chromobacterium violaceum*, *Francisella philomiragia*, and *Granulibacter bethesdensis*)
Acute Tuberculosis	Disseminated disease or miliary disease	Consider acute tuberculosis in critically ill patients with enigmatic acute respiratory distress syndrome, shock, or disseminated intravascular coagulation. This form often occurs among immunocompromised hosts such as those with HIV/AIDS

[a]*Some of these conditions may mimic at the time of presentation a picture of severe sepsis and thus are considered within the differential diagnosis of someone presenting with community-acquired SIRS/sepsis (see Table 1.2).*
[b]*Myxomas, TTP and the antiphospholipid syndrome may mimic acute bacterial endocarditis.*
[c]*Patients with a history of splenectomy or functional asplenia often need to have antibiotics available to be initiated as soon as fever or any symptoms consistent with an active infectious process. Patients with an episode of community-acquired sepsis and history of splenectomy often require chronic suppressive antibiotic therapy.*
[d]*Cases of sepsis associated with venous limb gangrene, symmetric peripheral gangrene and manifesting as acral skin necrosis or purpura fulminans (due to microcirculation thrombosis and natural anticoagulant failure) have been associated with meningococcal infection, pneumococcal infection, Escherichia coli, Capnocytophaga spp, disseminated tuberculosis, viral infections, and rickettsia.*

The presence of SIRS presents the possibility of a differential diagnosis of: (1) infectious causes, and (2) noninfectious causes. There are some clinical entities where physiologic changes in response noninfectious events such as pancreatitis, burns, or trauma are consistent with SIRS. There are two pathogenic pathways, which may result in SIRS (Fig. 1.1). Dysregulated and overwhelming systemic inflammation may result in response to exogenous microbial pathogen-associated molecular patterns (PAMPs) or by the release of endogenous cellular contents from damaged tissue or dying cells in the form of damage-associated molecular patterns (DAMPs).[5] In this context, exogenous PAMPs and endogenous DAMPs are then recognized by molecular receptors on cells of innate

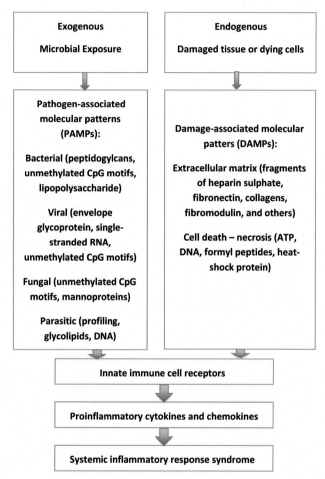

FIGURE 1.1   **Two pathogenic triggering pathways for the systemic inflammatory response syndrome.**

immune response (macrophages and polymorphonuclear cells). This group of receptors are termed pattern-recognition receptors and include the extracellular toll-like receptors or the intracellular nucleotide-binding oligomerization domain-like receptors (NOD), C-type lectin receptors, receptor for advanced glycation end products, or the retinoic acid-inducible-gene-1-like receptors.

The acute phase reactants are a group of molecular adaptations that may accompany sepsis. This group of proteins and inflammatory markers were named after the discovery of the C-reactive protein (so called due to the inflammatory changes induced by the pneumococcal C-polysaccharide) in the plasma during the acute phase of pneumococcal pneumonia.[7] These acute-phase proteins are induced by cytokines and other extracellular signaling molecules to contribute to defensive or adaptive capabilities. Several cytokines, particularly interleukin-6 stimulate the production of acute-phase proteins in response to infection. Some of them may be measured as markers of sepsis.[4]

HOSPITAL ACQUIRED SEPSIS

The incidence and severity of sepsis appear to be increasing in hospital settings. Some of the identified risk factors include a nosocomial infection, bacteremia, immunosuppression, advanced age, and community acquired pneumonia. Frequent causes of hospital-acquired sepsis include catheter-associated urinary tract infections, fungemia (ie, candidemia), bloodstream infections associated with vascular access, empyema, cholangitis, peritonitis, and severe and complicated *Clostridium difficile* infection.

COMMUNITY ACQUIRED SEPSIS

This broad group of conditions is characterized by the onset of SIRS associated with an infectious process with rapid progression to severe sepsis in the outpatient setting requiring prompt inpatient interventions to halt the progression of the sepsis cascade in order to improve clinical outcomes. Host factors may predispose some individuals to develop a particular condition such as terminal complement deficiencies associated with meningococcemia. Similarly, asplenic individuals may develop rapidly progressive community-acquired sepsis when exposed to encapsulated bacteria such as *S. pneumonia* or *Hemophilus influenza*, exposure to tickborne babesiosis, or a dog bite with inoculation of the bacterium *Capnocytophaga canimorsus*. Table 1.3 depicts some of the common causes of community-acquired sepsis.

REFERENCES

1. Del Casino VJ, Butterworth M, Davis G. The slippery geographies of polio. *Lancet Infect Dis* 2014;**14**:546–7.
2. Ochman H, Wilson AC. Evolution in bacteria: evidence for a universal substitution rate in cellular genomes. *J Mol Evol* 1987;**26**:74–86.
3. Blaser M. Stop the killing of beneficial bacteria. *Nature* 2011;**476**:393–4.
4. Klempner MS, Talbot EA, Lee SI, Zaki S, Ferraro MJ. Case 25-2010: a 24-year-old woman with abdominal pain and shock. *N Engl J Med* 2010;**363**(8):766–77.
5. Angus DC. The lingering consequences of sepsis: a hidden public health disaster? *J Am Med Assoc* 2010;**304**(16):1833–4.
6. Mohajer MA, Darouiche RO. Sepsis syndrome, bloodstream infections, and device-related infections. *Med Clin N Am* 2012;**96**:1203–23.
7. Gabay C, Kushner I. Acute-phase proteins and other systemic responses to inflammation. *N Engl J Med* 1999;**340**(6):448–53.

Chapter 2

Bloodstream Infections

DIAGNOSTIC APPROACH TO BLOODSTREAM INFECTIONS

Bloodstream infections include infective endocarditis, central venous catheter-associated bloodstream infections, primary bacteremia, and those with secondary bacteremia due to focal infections including abscesses, osteomyelitis, urinary tract infections, or pneumonia (Fig. 2.1). Bloodstream infection is a major cause of morbidity and mortality despite the availability of broad spectrum and effective antimicrobials and major advances in supportive care. Bacterial endocarditis accounts for approximately 3–8% of cases of bloodstream infections (see chapter: Neck and Thoracic Infections).

An infectious pathogen reach the bloodstream by direct invasion into blood vessels, via lymphatic vessels draining a focus of infection (ie, abscess), or through vascular devices such as needles of catheters. It may also occur without a clearly identifiable mechanism, for example, in some cases of complicated community-acquired *S. aureus* bacteremia.[1,2] The spleen is major immune organ for responding to invasive pathogens reaching the bloodstream. Sterilization and clearance of viable bacteria from the bloodstream and from the original source of infection is crucial in improving those physiological parameters of SIRS.[3] Beside source removal (eg, removal of an intravascular device; or surgical drainage of an intraabdominal abscess) and the institution of specific antimicrobial therapy, the goal of treating a patient with sepsis is to maintain cellular oxygenation via support of organ perfusion.

Blood cultures are usually obtained along with clinical investigations to search for a focus of infection and therefore provide specific antimicrobial therapy. Blood cultures should not be routinely ordered for adult patients with isolated fever or leucocytosis without considering factors such as the presence of systemic inflammatory response syndrome (SIRS) or the presence of chills, both of which raise the pretest probability of blood cultures yielding bacteremia in the right clinical setting.[1]

BACTEREMIA

This term refers to any true-positive blood culture, which reflects the presence of viable bacteria in the bloodstream.[2] The administration of antimicrobials prior to obtaining blood cultures reduces their sensitivity. In general, approximately

Core Concepts in Clinical Infectious Diseases (CCCID). http://dx.doi.org/10.1016/B978-0-12-804423-0.00002-0

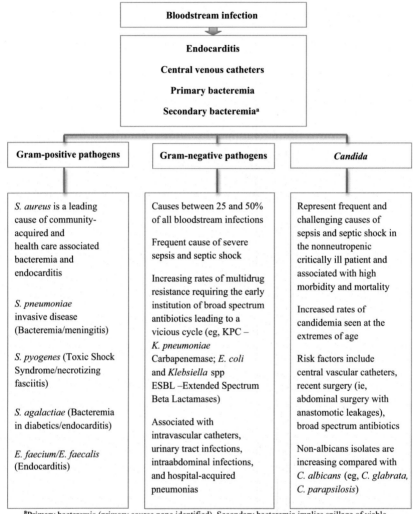

ᵃPrimary bacteremia (primary source none identified). Secondary bacteremia implies spillage of viable bacteria into the bloodstream from a focal infection such as a urinary tract infection, pneumonia, or abscess.

FIGURE 2.1   **Gram-negative, gram-positive, and *Candida* bloodstreams infections.**

4–7% of blood cultures obtained are reported positive, however, this may vary in different settings.[1] The presence of bacteremia induces an inflammatory response that is responsible of producing the symptoms of a bloodstream infection (ie, fever and chills).[1] The onset of SIRS associated with bacteremia has prognostic implications, although, its clinical significance varies with underlying illness and the source of the bacteremia.[3]

Gram-negative bacteremia, which often produce sepsis or septic shock associated with their lipopolysaccharide of their cell walls, were at some point the predominant organisms isolated in blood cultures in the hospital setting.[2] Currently, bacteremia due to gram-negative bacilli constitute approximately 25–50% of all causes of bloodstream infections and are important sources or morbidity and mortality given the increasing rates of antimicrobial resistance (Fig. 2.1). Gram-positive organisms including *S. aureus*, coagulase-negative staphylococci, and enterocci), and *Candida* species have become an important cause of bloodstream infections.[4] This trend is largely the result of increasing use of intravascular catheter devices. *S. aureus* is a leading cause of bloodstream infections in many settings[5] (Table 2.1). Some selected conditions associated with other gram-positive bacteremias are depicted in Table 2.2.

TABLE 2.1 Core Concepts in Bacteremia Caused by *S. aureus*[a]

Types	**Uncomplicated** (1) Endocarditis has been excluded; (2) no implanted prostheses are present; (3) follow-up blood cultures drawn 2–4 days after the initial set are sterile; (4) patient defervesce within 72 h of initiation of effective antibiotic therapy; and (5) no evidence of metastatic infection **Complicated** Usually manifested as continuous bacteremia and with evidence of metastatic infection
Associated complications	Left-sided endocarditis Right-sided endocarditis Vertebral osteomyelitis Epidural abscess Hematogenous osteomyelitis Subdural abscess Waterhouse–Friderichsen syndrome Mycotic aneurysm and stroke
Duration of therapy	*Overall recommendation*: 4–6 weeks of intravenous antibiotics *Uncomplicated bacteremia*: 14 days of effective intravenous antibiotics from the time of first negative blood culture *Complicated bacteremia*: 4–6 of effective intravenous antibiotics from the time of first negative blood culture *Often prolonged courses*: More than 6 weeks are indicated on the basis of clinical course and microbiologic criteria
Removal of source	Long-term catheters should be removed Short-term catheters including central lines should also be removed in most cases of suspected infection, particularly if the patient is developing sepsis/septic shock Surgical or percutaneous drainage of metastatic foci of infection (epidural abscess, empyema, liver abscess, or other)

[a]*Tong SYC, Davis JS, Eichenberger E, Holland TL, Fowler VG. Staphylococcus aureus infections: epidemiology, pathophysiology, clinical manifestations, and management. Clin Microb Rev 2015; 28(3):604–660.*

TABLE 2.2 Selected Clinical Syndromes Associated with Gram-Positive Bacteremias

Category	Organism(s)	Diseases/syndromes
Viridans group streptococci (VGS)	*Streptococcus mitis* group *Streptococcus mutans* group	Subacute bacterial endocarditis Aspiration Pneumonitis/empyema Pylephlebitis
Streptococcus pneumoniae[a]	Frequent serotypes (eg, 14, 6B, 19F, 23F)	Invasive Disease (Bacteremia, meningitis, endocarditis)
β-Hemolytic streptococci of groups other than A and B[b]	*Streptococcus dysgalactiae* subspecies equisimilis	Bacteremia secondary to skin and soft-tissue infections in older patients Septic arthritis, pneumonia, endocarditis, osteomyelitis, toxic shock syndrome
	Streptococcus anginosus group[c]	Intraabdominal infections in younger individual
Streptococcus pyogenes	Suppurative complications	Cellulitis/necrotizing fasciitis Septic arthritis, osteomyelitis, pneumonia Invasive disease (bacteremia, endocarditis, meningitis)
	Nonsuppurative complications	Rheumatic fever Scarlet fever Toxic shock syndrome Glomerulonephritis
Streptococcus agalactiae	Pregnancy	Urinary tract infections, amnionitis, chorioamnionitis, endometritis, and postpartum wound infections
	Neonates	Within first 7 days of birth, respiratory infection or neonatal sepsis
	Other adults	Late onset 3rd–4th week bacteremia, meningitis, osteomyelitis, septic arthritis, and cellulitis Bacteremia/cellulitis/septic arthritis, pneumonia, urinary tract infection
Enterococci	*Enterococcus faecalis* *Enterococcus faecium*	Endocarditis[d] Intrabdominal Infections Bacteremia
		Most frequent species with Vancomycin resistance
Previously nutritionally variant streptococci	*Abiotrophia* spp *Granulicatella* spp	Bacteremia Endovascular infections (ie, mycotic aneurysm Skin-soft tissue infections Endocarditis Pancreatic abscess Otitis media Conjunctivitis

TABLE 2.2 Selected Clinical Syndromes Associated with Gram-Positive Bacteremias (*cont.*)

Category	Organism(s)	Diseases/syndromes
Coagulase negative staphylococci	*Staphylococcus epidermidis/ hominis*	Endocarditis among patients with hemodialysis vascular access infection(s)
	Staphylococcus lugdunensis Staphylococcus schleiferi[e]	Bacteremia Endocarditis postvasectomy Metastatic infection

[a]*Invasive disease refers to bacteremia or presence of the bacteria in sterile tissues or spaces.*
[b]*The nongroup A or B, hemolytic streptococci are frequently normal inhabitants of the oropharynx, skin, and gastrointestinal and genitourinary tracts (Broyles LN, Beneden CV, Beall B, Facklam R, Shewmaker PL, Malpiedi P, et al. Population-based study of invasive disease due to β-hemolytic streptococci of groups other than A and B. Clin Infect Dis 2009;48:706–712).*
[c]*Streptococcus anginosus group consists of:* S. anginosus, S. constellatus, S. constellatus *subspecies* constellatus, S. constellatus *subspecies* pharynges.
[d]*Streptococcus bovis has been associated with colon carcinoma. However, unexplained enterococci bacteremia is in clinical practice more frequently associated with colon polyps and colon carcinoma. Clostridium septicum has also been associated with colon carcinoma. Unexplained S. agalactiae in a female patient may indicate intrauterine neoplasias such as endometrial carcinoma.*
[e]*Of the coagulase-negative staphylococci,* Staphylococcus lugdunensis *and* S. schleiferi *can cause severe complications due to metastatic disease. A single culture of* S. lugdunensis *is clinically significant.*

ENDOVASCULAR INFECTIONS

The term "endovascular infection" is often used to refer to a condition where there is continuous bacteremia despite the institution of adequate antimicrobial therapy. Although *S. aureus* may use vascular endothelial cells to thrive and produce a true endovascular infection, this term should be reserved for infection of the wall of large vessels belonging to the systemic, pulmonary, or venous system and often producing aneursyms, pseudoaneurysms, or even arteriovenous fistulae.[6,7] Common bacterial pathogens that cause endovascular infections include *Salmonella*, *Abiotrophia*,[8] and *Granulicatella* species. *Mycobacterium bovis* in the form of BCG infusion for bladder carcinomas has been also associated with endovascular infections. In this context, infection of the endocardium/ cardiac valves as part of endocarditis should be considered within the spectrum of endovascular infections (see chapter: Neck and Thoracic Infections). In summary, although continuous or persistent bacteremia despite institution of therapy is a feature of endovascular infections, this group of infections imply infection of the wall of a large vessel (endarteritis) or the endocardium (endocarditis).

FUNGEMIA

Candidemia is the fourth most common bloodstream infection reported from intensive care units, but in population-based studies it is reported as the seventh to tenth most common bloodstream infection.[4] Mortality increases to up to 40%

TABLE 2.3 Core Concepts in Bloodstream Infections Associated with *Candida* Species[a]

Overall management issues	Empiric therapy with an echinocandin should be initiated pending species identification and susceptibility Antifungal therapy can be narrowed to fluconazole if species identified as *Candida parapsilosis, Candida tropicalis, Candida lusitaniae*. Antifungal therapy with an echinocandin should be continued for cases of *Candida glabrata* and *Candida krusei*. Voriconazole may be an alternate oral treatment for *C. krusei* if susceptibility testing has been performed on the isolate. All patients with candidemia should undergo an ophthalmological exam Consider empiric antifungal therapy in patients with sepsis and multiple risk factors for invasive candidemia (recent abdominal surgery, parenteral nutrition, exposure to broad-spectrum antibiotics, known colonization with *Candida* spp. in multiple nonsterile sites) especially if these patients have not responded to antibacterial therapy
Associated complications (hematogenous spread)	Endophtalmitis/chorioretinitis/vitritis Endocarditis (large vegetations) Meningitis Osteomyelitis
Duration of therapy	Clearance of candidemia must be documented by repeat blood cultures Duration of antifungal therapy should be 14 days from the time of first negative cultures
Removal of source	All intravascular catheters should be removed including implantable tunneled catheters, dialysis catheters, etc. For patients with dialysis catheters, the catheter can be removed following dialysis (unless patient has septic shock or new organ dysfunction in which case it should be removed immediately) with a new temporary dialysis catheter inserted just prior to the next dialysis treatment

[a]*Other fungi that may be identified on blood cultures include:* Cryptococcus, Histoplasma, Coccidioides *and other dimorphic fungi; and molds such as* Fusarium.

even when patients receive adequate antifungal therapy. Core concepts on the diagnostic approach and management of fungemias are noted in Table 2.3.

CATHETER-ASSOCIATED BLOODSTREAM INFECTIONS

Many bloodstream infections are linked to intravascular access devices. Among them, central-line-associated bloodstream infection (CLABSI) is associated with increased length of hospital stay and increased inpatient mortality. The term catheter-related blood-stream infection (CRBSI) encompasses not only

CLABSI but also long-term indwelling catheters used for parenteral nutrition, chemotherapy, outpatient antibiotic infusions, or other drugs for chronic medical conditions (eg, intravenous immune globulin).[2] CLABSI terminology is used mostly for surveillance purposes, whereas CRBSI is used clinically when diagnosing or treating patients. The definition of CRBSI includes the presence of bacteremia (with at least one blood culture obtained from a peripheral vein percutaneously) or fungemia in a patient who has an intravascular catheter, with clinical signs of infection (fever, chills, hypotension), and the absence of other source of infection. Other criteria that assist clinicians in diagnosing CRBSI and thus, the likely need of catheter removal, is a positive quantitative or semiquantitative catheter tip culture, quantitative blood culture, or a differential time to positivity (blood culture from drawn from catheter becomes positive at least 2 h earlier compared with peripherally obtained blood culture).

Long-term catheters should be removed in cases of bloodstream infections with *S. aureus, Pseudomonas aeruginosa, Fusarium, Candida*, or nontuberculous mycobacteria regardless of disease severity. Short-term catheters including central lines should also be removed in most cases of suspected infection, particularly if the patient is developing sepsis/septic shock.

REFERENCES

1. Coburn B, Morris AM, Tomlinson G, Detsky AS. Does this adult patient with suspected bacteremia require blood cultures? *J Am Med Assoc* 2012;**308**(5):502–11.
2. Mohajer MA, Darouiche RO. Sepsis syndrome, bloodstream infections, and device-related infections. *Med Clin North Am* 2012;**96**:1203–23.
3. Rangel-Frausto MS, Pittet D, Costigan M, Hwang T, Davis CS, Wenzel RP. The natural history of the systemic inflammatory response syndrome (SIRS): a prospective study. *JAMA* 1995;**273**(2):117–23.
4. Kullberg BJ, Arendrup MC. Invasive candidiasis. *N Engl J Med* 2015;**373**(15):1445–56.
5. Holland TL, Arnold C, Fowler VG. Clinical management of *Staphylococcus aureus* bacteremia. *J Am Med Assoc* 2014;**312**.(13):1330–41.
6. Olsen EGJ. Endovascular infections. *Postrad Med J* 1989;**65**:127–8.
7. Senn L, Entenza JM, Greub G, Jaton K, Wenger A, Bille J, et al. Bloodstream and endovascular infections due to *Abiotrophia defectiva* and *Granulicatella* species. *BMC Infect Dis* 2006;**6**:9.
8. Franco-Paredes C, Workowski K. Infective endocarditis-endarteritis complicating coarctation of the aorta. *Am J Med* 2002;**112**:590–2.

Chapter 3

Central Nervous System Syndromes

DIAGNOSTIC APPROACH AND DIFFERENTIAL DIAGNOSIS OF MAJOR NEUROLOGIC SYNDROMES

Evaluation of the Cerebrospinal Fluid

Cells within the central nervous system (CNS) are capable of producing an immune response against invading pathogens. More importantly, the brain is protected by the blood–brain barrier. Microbial pathogens may access the CNS by penetrating the blood–brain barrier or via the olfactory and/or trigeminal nerves. Penetration of the blood–brain barrier is the most common route of invasion into the CNS of bacterial pathogens via a transcellular route, paracellular route, or through a "Trojan-horse" mechanism by inflammatory cells such as monocytes[1] (Table 3.1). The trigeminal and olfactory nerves are also recognized portal of entry for many viruses, protozoa, and fungi, as well as for some bacterial pathogens. The cerebrospinal fluid (CSF) plays an essential function in maintaining the homeostasis of the neuraxis in terms of electrolyte balance, circulation of active molecules, elimination of catabolites, and inflammatory responses to infection.

The CSF circulates rostro-caudally surrounding the subarachnoid space of the brain parenchyma and spinal cord; and the cerebral ventricles. In addition to its role of hydromechanical protection of the CNS, CSF performs a central function in brain development and regulation of parenchymal interstitial fluid homeostasis and neuronal functioning.[1] In regular conditions, CSF is produced in the choroid plexus at a rate of 20 mL/h to a volume of about 125–150 mL of which approximately 20% is contained in the ventricular system and the rest percolates throughout subarachnoid space surrounding the neuraxis. The CSF is continuously reabsorbed in the arachnoid villi in the lumen of the intracranial venous sinuses (finger-like endothelium-lined protrusions of the outer layer of the arachnoid through the duramater layer). CSF communicates with interstitial fluid via the Virchow–Robin perivascular spaces.

Therefore, the evaluation of the CSF is one of the most reliable laboratory assessments in clinical medicine when considering selected major clinical infectious diseases syndromes of the CNS such as meningitis and encephalitis (Table 3.2).

Core Concepts in Clinical Infectious Diseases (CCCID). http://dx.doi.org/10.1016/B978-0-12-804423-0.00003-2

TABLE 3.1 Invasion Pathways of Pathogens Penetrating the Central Nervous System[a]

Type of mechanism[b]	Examples
Transcellular penetration of brain microvascular endothelial cells (BBB)	*Escherichia coli* *S. pneumoniae* *Listeria monocytogenes* *Streptococcus agalactiae* (GBS) *Cryptococcus neoformans*
Paracellular penetration of microvascular endothelial cells (BBB)	*H. influenzae* *N. meningitidis* *Cryptococcus neoformans*
Trojan horse of brain microvascular endothelial cells (BBB)	*Burkholderia pseudomallei* *Listeria monocytogenes* *Cryptococcus neoformans*
Exogenous	*Staphylococcus epidermidis* or *Pseudomonas aeruginosa* infection of a cerebrospinal shunt[c] Nosocomial meningitis after a neurosurgical procedures *Streptococcus pneumoniae* among individuals with skull base fractures Epidural injection of corticosteroids (methylprednisolone) contaminated with *Exserhilum rostratum*[d]

Cranial nerves	*Olfactory nerve* *Bacterial* • Bypasses the cellular barriers of the CNS and provides a direct portal from the nasal cavity to the olfactory bulb by *B. pseudomallei* and possibly *N. meningitidis* in the African belt *Viral* • Herpesviruses • Influenza A • Paramyxovirues (Nipah, hendra) • Eastern, Western, and Venezuelan Equine Encephalitis following aerosol exposure • Rabies *Parasitic* • *Naegleria fowleri* • *Balamuthia mandrilaris* *Trigeminal nerve* *Bacterial* (*B. pseudomallei, L. monocytogenes*) *Viral* • Herpes viruses *Fungal* • Rhinocerebral mucormycosis

BBB, Blood-brain barrier; CSF, cerebrospinal fluid.

*a*It is important to consider prion diseases within the infectious disease spectrum. This group of infectious agents is composed of protein, which can fold in multiple structurally distinct ways, self-propagates, and transmits its conformation to other prion proteins. These abnormal proteins cause the transmissible spongiform encephalopathies. They tend to produce an encephalopathy with rapid progression to dementia. (Rinne ML, McGinnis SM, Samuels MA, Katz JT, Loscalzo J. A startling decline. N Engl J Med 2012;**366**:836–842).

*b*Dando SJ, Mackay-Sim A, Norton R, Currie BJ, St. John JA, Ekberg JAK, et al. Pathogens penetrating the central nervous system: Infection pathways and the cellular and molecular mechanisms of invasion. Clin. Microb. Rev 2014;**27**(4):691–713.

*c*Most common causes of CSF shunts infections include Staphylococcus aureus, Propionibacterium acnes and its rate of infection varies from 1 to 18% in different reports. Infected cerebrospinal shunts should be removed temporarily with external ventricular drains and patients treated with antibiotics before reinsertion of new shunt ensuring sterility of the CSF (Mohajer MA, Darouiche RO. Sepsis syndrome, bloodstream infections, and device-related infections. Med Clin North Am 2012;**96**:1203–1223).

*d*Kauffman CA, Pappas PG, Patterson TF. Fungal infections associated with contaminated methylprednisolone injections. N Engl J Med 2013;**368**(26):2495–2499.

TABLE 3.2 Differential Diagnosis of Cerebrospinal Fluid Analysis

Type	Features	Differential diagnosis
Type 1	WBC > 500 but usually less than 1000 predominanty polymorphonuclear cells Hypoglycorrachia (less than two-thirds of systemic glucose) Elevated Protein (>60 mg/dL)	Acute Bacterial Meningitis • *S. pneumoniae* • *N. meningitidis* • *L. monocytogenes* • *H. influenza* Necrotizing encephalitis due to Naegleria fowlerii Parameningeal process (subdural empyema)
Type 2	WBC> 500 predominantly mononuclear cells (Lymphocytes) Hypoglycorrachia (less than two-thirds of systemic glucose)[a] Elevated protein (>60 mg/dL)	Tuberculous meningitis *Fungal* C. neoformans or Cryptococcus gattii; Cocciodiodomycosis, Histoplasma capsulatum Carcinomatous meningitis Sarcoidosis *Viral meningitis* Mumps, Lymphocytic choriomeningitis virus, HSV-2 meningitis
Type 3	WBC > 50 predominantly mononuclear cells Normal glucose and normal protein (or slightly elevated protein)	*Viral meningitis/aseptic meningitis* Echovirus, coxsackievirus Acute HIV Drug-induced meningitis Viral encephalitis[b,c]
Type 4	WBC and RBC normal Elevated protein[d]	Guillain–Barré Syndrome[e]

WBC, White blood cell counts; PMN, polymorphonuclear cells; GBS, Guillain–Barré syndrome.
[a]*Other cause of reduced glucose in CSF is subarachnoid hemorrhage.*
[b]*Herpes simplex encephalitis may also have abundant red cells.*
[c]*Xantochromia is a yellowish discoloration of the CSF supernatant due to bilirubin and its causes include: (1) subarachnoid hemorrhage, (2) methemoglobin in CSF, (3) high-protein in CSF > 1500 mg/L by the binding of protein with bilirubin; and (4) systemic hyperbilirrubinemia.*
[d]*Levels of CSF protein are usually higher in bacterial meningitis compared with aseptic meningitis. At a cut off value of 100 mg/L, the sensitivity and specificity for distinguishing bacterial from aseptic meningitis are 82 and 98%, respectively (Venkatesh B, Scott P, Ziegenfuss M. Cerebrospinal fluid in critical illness. Crit Care Resusc 2000;**2**:42–54).*
[e]*Albumino-cytologic dissociation is present in less than 50% of patients with GBS.*

Meningitis

Many microbes can invade the CNS and may potentially cause meningitis. Meningitis, or inflammation of the meninges, can be pyogenic, which is associated with common bacterial pathogens or aseptic (when no organism is isolated or identified) (Table 3.3). In certain circumstances, acute meningitis can be clinically indistinguishable from acute encephalitis (Table 3.4), which refers to the inflammatory process of the brain parenchyma leading to neurologic dysfunction.

TABLE 3.3 Differential Diagnosis of Meningitis by Infectious Pathogen

Category	Etiologies	Core concepts
Infectious	Bacterial[a]	S. pneumonia L. monocytogenes H. influenza T. pallidum B. burdorgferi[b]
	Viral	Enteroviruses[c] • Coxsackie • ECHO HIV EBV, CMV West Nile virus[d]
	Fungal	Cryptococcal (C. neoformans, C. gattii) Coccidiodomycosis (C. immitis) Histoplasma Aspergillus fumigatus
	Parasitic	Acanthamoeba Angystrongyloides cantonensis Gnathostoma spirigerum Trypanosoma brucei rhodesiense (Human African trypanosomiasis – HAT) Trypanosoma cruzi (Chagas disease)[e]
Inflammatory	Behcet's disease Vogt–Koyanagi–Harada syndrome Systemic lupus Erythematosus	
Drug-induced	NSAIDs Intravenous immune globulin Antibiotics (cotrimoxazole)	Patients symptoms gradually improve after removal of inciting drug
Neoplastic	Lymphoma Breast carcinoma	Lymphomatous meningitis Carcinomatous meningitis

[a]The pathogenic sequence of bacterial neurotropism include four stages: (1) colonization or mucosal invasion; (2) intravascular survival; (3) crossing or entering the blood–brain barrier; and (4) survival within the cerebrospinal fluid. In order to achieve its goal to reach and thrive in the CNS, pathogens have adapted through molecular ingenuity such as by the use of IgA protease secretion, inducing ciliostasis in the respiratory epithelium, production of adhesive pili, and evasion of the alternative pathway of the complement (Quagliarello V, Scheld WM. Bacterial meningitis: pathogenesis, pathophysiology, and progress. N Engl J Med 1992;327(12):864–872).
[b]Lyme disease follows a subacute course compared with viral/aseptic meningitis. Lymphocytic choriomeningitis virus should be suspected when there is a history of exposure to rodents excreta.
[c]Acute viral meningitis is mostly caused by group B Coxsackievirus and echovirus types. Numerous serotypes have implicated as causes of encephalitis including Coxsackievirus types A9, B2, and B5, Echovirus types 6 and 9, and Enterovirus 71. (Rotbart HA. Enteroviral infections of the central nervous system. Clin Infect Dis 1995;20:971–981).
[d]Gould EA. West Nile virus: don't underestimate its persistence. J Infect Dis 2010;201:1.
[e]Human African trypanosomiasis or "sleeping sickness" and Chagas disease are characterized as meningoencephalitis.

TABLE 3.4 Differential Diagnosis of Encephalitis[a]

Infectious[b]	Viral Herpes simplex virus Varicella–Zoster virus Herpes B CMV Mumps Rabies	Predominantly affects parenchymal grey matter with perivascular and parenchymal infiltration of inflammatory cells and neuronophagia
	Arthropod-borne virus encephalitis	
	Flavivirus Japanese encephalitis, West Nile Virus encephalitis, St. Louis Encephalitis	West Nile virus and Japanese encephalitis viruses may produce acute flaccid paralysis, tremor, myoclonus
		St. Louis encephalitis causes tremors of eyelids, tongue, lips, and extremities, cranial nerve palsies
	Togavirus Eastern equine encephalitis (EEE)	EEE may be associated with lesions in basal ganglia in MRI
	Bunyavirus La Crosse encephalitis	La Crosse encephalitis may mimic HSV-1 temporal encephalitis
	Powasan Virus	
	Coltivirus Colorado Tick Fever	
	Bacterial Rickettsia Borreliosis Mycoplasma pneumoniae Treponema species	Rocky Mountain spotted fever (RMSF), ehrlichiosis, and anaplasmosis may mimick viral encephalitis
	Tropheryma whippleii	Whipple disease may manifest as encephalitis with supranuclear gaze palsy, cranial nerve abnormalities, fever, seizures, ataxia, myorhythmia, and sensory deficits[c]
	Listeria monocytogenes	Rhombencephalitis
	Bartonella henselleae	Retinitis
	Protozoan Balamuthia mandrillaris Naegleria fowleri Acanthamoeba Toxoplasma gondii	Naegleria fowleri produces a rapidly progressive necrotizing encephalitis while Balamuthia and Acanthamoeba may produce more subacute granulomatous meningoencephalitis
	Helminthic Baylisascaris procynosis	Exposure to raccoon feces

TABLE 3.4 Differential Diagnosis of Encephalitis[a] (*cont.*)

Postinfectious	*Postviral* Coxsackie virus EBV CMV Influenza	It is a disease predominantly affecting white matter, with perivenular inflammation and demyelination often termed acute disseminated encephalomyelitis (ADEM)
Autoimmune	Anti-NMDA Antivoltage gated potassium channel	Possible association with infections (ie, *Mycoplasma*)
Paraneoplastic (antineuronal-antibody-associated paraneoplastic disorders)[d]	Anti-Hu	Paraneoplastic encephalomyelitis (small-cell lung cancer, neuroblastoma, prostate cancer)
	Anti-Hu Anti-Yo	Paraneoplastic cerebellar degeneration (ovarian, breast, and lung carcinomas)
	Antivoltage gated calcium channels	Lambert–Eaton myasthenic syndrome (small cell lung carcinoma)
	Anti-Ma1	Brain-stem encephalitis (lung carcinomas)
	Anti Ma2	Limbic brain-stem encephalitis (testicular cancer)

[a]*Tunkel AR, Glaser CA, Bloch KC, Sejvar JJ, Marra CM, Roos KL, et al. The management of encephalitis: clinical practice guidelines by the Infectious Diseases Society of America.* Clin Infect Dis 2008;**47**:303–327.
[b]*It is also useful from a clinical standpoint and to consider in the differential diagnosis regional forms of encephalitis: (1) limbic: paraneoplastic origin, anti-NMDA or anti-voltage gated potassium channel; (2) temporal lobe (HSV-1); (3) rhombencephalitis (enterovirus 71,* Listeria monocytogenes HSV-1, HHV-6, West Nile virus, rabies virus, melioidosis, bulbar poliomyelitis) (Jubelt B, Mihai C, Li Tm, Veerapaneni P. Curr Neurol Neurosci Rep 2011;**11**:543–552).
[c]*Ghezzi A, Zaffaroni M. Neurological manifestations of gastrointestinal disorders, with particular reference to the differential diagnosis of multiple sclerosis.* Neurol Sci 2001;**22**:S117–S122.
[d]*Darnell RB, Posner JB. Paraneoplastic syndromes involving the nervous system.* N Engl J Med 2003;**349**(16):1543–1554.

Bacterial meningitis remains as an important cause of morbidity and mortality despite the advent of effective antimicrobials. In fact suboptimal outcomes may occur despite microbiologic cure as a result of the inflammatory response to the pathogenic agent. Therefore, most efforts should be placed toward preventing this condition in the first use and in this context, the use of conjugate vaccines against *Hemophilus influenzae* and *Streptococcus pneumoniae* have reduced substantially the burden of disease associated with meningitis by offering important protection to vaccinated individuals; and through herd immunity by reducing colonization and likely household transmission.

TABLE 3.5 Predisposing Conditions Leading to Brain Abscess[a]

Predisposing conditions	Infectious agents
Paranasal sinusitis[b]	*Streptococcus* spp. and *Prevotella* spp.
Otitis media or otomastoiditis	*Streptococcus* spp. (anaerobic and aerobic), *Bacteroides* and *Prevotella*
Dental infections/abscess	Mixed oral bacteria such as Fusobacterium, Actinomyces, Bacteroides, and *Streptococcus* spp.
HIV/AIDS	Toxoplasmosis, *Nocardia*, *Listeria monocytogenes*, *Cryptococcus neoformans*
Acute bacterial endocarditis	*S. aureus* *Streptococcus viridans*
Penetrating trauma or neurosurgery	*Pseudomonas, Enterobacteriaceae, Clostridium* spp., *S. aureus*

[a]*Brouwer MC, Tunkel AR, McKhann II GM, van den Beek D. Brain abscess.* N Engl J Med 2014;**371**(5):447–456; Darouiche RO. Spinal epidural abscess. N. Engl. J Med 2006;**355**(19):2012–2020.
[b]*Paranasal sinusitis may be associated with suppurative intracranial infection including meningitis, intracranial abscess, subdural empyema, epidural abscess, cavernous sinus thrombosis, and thrombosis of other dural sinuses requiring a high index of suspicion (Osborn MK, Steinberg JP. Subdural empyema and other suppurative complications of paranasal sinusitis.* Lancet Infect Dis 2007;**7**:62–67).

Encephalitis

This syndrome is characterized by inflammation of the brain parenchyma that presents with altered level of consciousness, focal neurologic deficits (ie, seizures), and fever is termed encephalitis. Many pathogens may be associated with encephalitis[2] (Table 3.4). The clinical features of encephalitis may vary by causal pathogen, degree of parenchymal involvement and its location (temporal lobe, limbic, brainstem, or other locations) and host factors.

TABLE 3.6 Concomitant Lung-Brain Infectious Syndromes

Category	Specific pathogen
Bacterial	Nocardiosis
Mycobacterial	*Mycobacterium tuberculosis*
	Non-tuberculous Mycobacteria (NTM) such as *Mycobacterium abscessus*
Fungal	Blastomycosis Aspergillosis Histoplasmosis Coccidiodomycosis Cryptococcosis
Malignant	Nonsmall cell lung carcinoma (adenocarcinoma, squamous cell carcinoma)

Brain Abscess

In some patients, and depending on particular predisposing factors, bacteria, fungi, or parasitic infections may enter the brain parenchyma to cause an abscess or multiple abscesses (Table 3.5). The resulting clinical syndromes depend on the location of the abscess and the predisposing condition leading to its occurrence. Often, it is important to consider the possibility of a combination of lung infection and brain infection manifesting mostly as brain abscess (Table 3.6). It is important to consider infectious pathogens associated with cerebrovascular events since considering this diagnostic possibility provide clues to the specific diagnosis and management of some infectious pathogens of the CNS (Table 3.7).

TABLE 3.7 Strokes in the Setting of Central Nervous System Infections (Meningitis or Encephalitis)[a]

Category[b]	Specific pathogen	Disease manifestation
Viral[c]	Varicella-Zoster Virus[d]	Large vessel granulomatous angiitis (acute hemiplegia after contralateral trigemninal zoster in adults) or postvaricella arteriopathy in children Transient ischemic attacks Ischemic and hemorrhagic infarcts Subarachnoid Hemorrhage Arterial ectasia Multifocal VZV vasculopathy Temporal arteritis mimicking giant cell arteritis
	HIV	Ischemic and hemorrhagic infarcts
	Hepatitis C	Strokes associated with hypercoagulability
Mycobacterial	Mycobacterium Tuberculosis Mycobacterium abscessus	Basilar meningitis leading to inflammatory vasculitis usually of circle of Willis vasculature
Other bacterial	Brucella mellitensis/ abortus	Basilar meningitis leading to inflammatory vasculitis usually of Circle of Willis vasculature
Treponemal	Treponema pallidum	Frequently affecting the posterior circulation (eg, Parinaud syndrome and caused by two pathogenic forms: endarteritis obliterans of medium and large arteris (ie, Heubner arteritis) and Hissl-Alzheimer arteritis affecting small arterial vessels[e]

(Continued)

TABLE 3.7 Strokes in the Setting of Central Nervous System Infections (Meningitis or Encephalitis)[a] (cont.)

Category[b]	Specific pathogen	Disease manifestation
Fungal[f]	*Yeasts*	
	Cryptococcus spp *Candida spp* *Histoplasma capsulatum* *Coccidioides immitis* *Penicillium marneffei*	Cerebral ischemia from septic emboli or inflammatory vasculitis associated with basilar meningitis
	Molds	
	Aspergillus fumigatus *Fusarium species* *Mucor circinelloides*	Cerebral infarcts and mycotic aneurysms[g]
	Scedosporium apiospermum *Scedosporium prolificans*	Cerebral infarcts
	Dematiaceous mold	
	Cladophialophora bantiana *Ochroconis gallopava*	Cerebral infarcts
	Exserohillum rostratum	Cerebral infarct and mycotic aneurysms
Parasitic	*Schistosoma japonicum*	Cerebrovascular events
	Schistosoma mansoni *Schistosoma hematobium*	Spinal cord infarcts
	Gnathostoma spinigerium *Angiostrongylus cantonensis*	Cerebrovascular events (associated with meningitis in the setting of visceral larva migrans)

[a]*Fugate JE, Lyons JL, Thakur KT, Smith BR, Hedley-Whyte ET, Mateen FJ. Infectious causes of stroke. Lancet Infect Dis 2014;***14**:*869–880. It is important to consider that infectious endocarditis may be frequently linked to embolic strokes; and often dilated cardiomyopathies secondary to a viral myocarditis or Chagasic cardiomyopathy (Chagas disease caused by* Trypanosoma cruzi*) may lead to embolic strokes*
[b]*The posterior reversible encephalopathy (PRES) is a variant of hypertensive encephalopathy mainly involving the posterior areas of the brain. It is essential to distinguish this syndrome from cerebral ischemia. Some of the triggers of PRES may be drugs used in the management of infectious diseases including interferon-alpha, flucytosine (5-FC) for the treatment of cryptococcal meningitis or drugs used for immunosuppression including cyclosporine or tacrolimus. In addition, PRES is sometimes reported in the setting of HIV/AIDS (Mirza A. Posterior reversible encephalopathy syndrome: a variant of hypertensive encephalopathy. J Clin Neurosci 2006;***13**:*590–595).*
[c]*Infection due to Parvovirus B19 has been associated with strokes in patients with Sickle cell disease (Hemoglobin SS) but not meningitis or encephalitis concomitantly with stroke.*
[d]*Nagel MA, Gilden D. Complications of Varicella Zoster virus reactivation. Curr Treat Options Neurol 2013;***15**:*439–453.*
[e]*McCarthy M, Rosengart A, Schuetz AN, Kontoyiannis DP, Walsh TJ. Mold infections of the central nervous system. N Engl J Med 2014;***371**(12):*150–159.*
[f]*Bauerle J, Zitsmann A, Egger K, Meckel S, Weiller C, Harloff A. The great imitator – still today! A case of meningovascular syphilis affecting the posterior circulation. J Stroke Cerebrovasc Dis 2015;***24**(1): e1–e3.*
[g]*Mycotic aneurysm are caused by infection of the* vaso vasorum *(arterial wall) of intracranial blood vessels with secondary risk of stroke if it ruptures.*

TABLE 3.8 Differential Diagnosis of Ascending Paralysis Including Infectious Causes

Disease	Etiology	Core concepts
Guillian–Barré syndrome	Autoimmune	No ataxia, days to weeks of progression of ascending paralysis, and mild sensory loss
Tick paralysis[a]	*Dermacentor andersoni* *Dermacentor variabilis* *Ixodes holocyclus*[b]	Rapidly progressive ascending paralysis that affects mostly children and associated with paresthesias and leg weakness without fever. Patient has ataxia, difficulty walking with frequent falls and no sensory loss
Spinal cord lesions	Neoplasias, metastasis, epidural abscess	Sensory loss may be present, Babinsky present, Gradual or abrupt onset depending on the etiology. No ataxia
Viral	Poliomyelitis Coxsackievirus West Nile Virus Japanese Encephalitis Virus Tickborne Encephalitis Virus Enterovirus 71 Coxsackievirus	Present with fever and meningismus, ataxia, and ascending paralysis and elevated protein in cerebrospinal fluid

[a]*Tick paralysis is a neurologic syndrome that may mimic other neurologic conditions and it is caused by a neurotoxin produced by an attached and engorged tick (ie, Dermacentor variabilis). Other conditions that should be considered in the differential diagnosis include botulism, myasthenia gravis, periodic paralysis, electrolyte disorders, porphyria, insecticide poisoning, solvent inhalation, and hysterical paralysis (Felz MW, Davis Smith C, Swift TR. A six-year-old girl with tick paralysis. N Engl J Med 2000;**342**(2):90–94.*
[b]*Neurotoxin produced by Ixodes holocyclus tick interferes with the release of acetylcholine at the neuromuscular junction similar to the effect of botulinum toxin.*

MAJOR INFECTIOUS DISEASES AFFECTING THE SPINAL CORD, NERVE ROOTS, AND PERIPHERAL NERVES

The differential diagnosis of ascending paralysis is depicted in Table 3.8. The combination of areflexic paralysis with albumin-cytologic dissociation (normal cell counts and elevated protein) characterizes the Guillain–Barré syndrome (GBS). There are different clinical syndromes associated with this condition affecting the peripheral nerves or cranial nerves. The immune-pathogenesis of the GBS suggests that this syndrome encompasses a group of peripheral-nerve disorders. Each disorder is characterized by different underlying pathophysiology, by the distribution of weakness in the limbs or cranial nerve innervated muscles. In more than two-thirds of cases, there is a history of a preceding respiratory or gastrointestinal infectious process triggering an autoimmune response that translates into specific nerve affection depending on the location (cranial nerve versus peripheral nerves; and axonal versus myelin damage) (Table 3.9).

TABLE 3.9 Infectious Causes (Triggers) of the Guillain–Barré Syndrome

Subtypes and variants	Infectious agent triggering GBS	Antibody markers
Acute inflammatory demyelinating polyneuropathy	Cytomegalovirus (CMV) Epstein-Barr virus (EBV) Varicella-Zoster virus (VZV) HIV *Mycoplasma pneumonia* Hepatitis E Influenza Chikungunya	None identified
Acute motor axonal neuropathy • More or less extensive forms (acute motor-sensory axonal neuropathy and acute motor-conduction-block neuropathy) • Pharyngeal-cervical –brachial weakness	*Campylobacter jejuni*	GM-1, GD1a, GT1a[a]
Miller-Fisher syndrome[b] • Incomplete forms (acute ataxic neuropathy and acute ophtalmoparesis) • CNS variant: Bickerstaff's brainstem encephalitis	*Campylobacter jejuni* *Haemophilus influenzae*	GQ1b, GT1a

[a]*G refers to one of the four Gangliosides (GM1, GD1a, GT1a, and GQ1b) and the second letter (M, D, T, and Q) refer to the number of their sialic acids in the molecule where M, D, T, and Q represent mono, di, tri, and quadri-sialosyl groups.*
[b]*Miller–Fisher syndrome affecting cranial nerves should be distinguished from botulism, Wernicke's encephalopathy, myasthenia gravis, and brainstem stroke (Yuki N, Hartung HP. Guillain-Barré Syndrome. N Engl J Med 2012;366(24):2294–2304).*

There is a broad differential diagnosis when considering infectious causes of myelitis and spinal cord disorders (Table 3.10), peripheral neuropathies (Table 3.11), and toxin-mediated syndromes of the nervous system (tetanus and botulism) and its differential diagnosis and diagnostic approach (Table 3.12).

TABLE 3.10 Infectious Causes of Spinal Cord Diseases[a]

Disease	Etiology	Core concepts
Bacterial with associated spondylodiskitis	Bacterial	Tuberculosis[b] (Pott's diseases)
		Neurobrucellosis
		Pyogenic epidural abscess (eg, *S. aureus*) associated with bacteremia

TABLE 3.10 Infectious Causes of Spinal Cord Diseases[a] (cont.)

Disease	Etiology	Core concepts
Spinal cord vasculopathy caused by an infectious pathogen	Bacterial	Meningovascular syphilis
	Parasitic	*Schistosoma mansoni* and *S. haematobium*
Neuroborreliosis	*Borrelia burdorgferi*	Classic triad includes peripheral facial nerve palsies, aseptic meningitis, and painful radiculitis
Transverse myelitis[c]	Infectious	*Herpesviruses*[c] CMV Epstein–Barr virus (EBV) VZV HHV-6 Enterovirus HIV
		Bacterial Mycoplasma Borrelia burdorgferi
Chronic spastic paralysis	HTLV-1[d]	*Retroviruses* HTLV-1 HTLV-3 (HIV)
Acute flaccid paralysis	Viral	*Picornavirus* Poliovirus Coxackievirus A and B Echoviruses Enterovirus 71
		Flaviviruses West Nile Virus Japanese Enchepalitis Virus Tick-borne encephalitis virus
		Rhabdoviridae Rabies virus
Transverse Myelitis combined with Radiculitis	Viral	Herpesviruses HSV-1, HSV-2 CMV EBV VZV

(*Continued*)

TABLE 3.10 Infectious Causes of Spinal Cord Diseases[a] (cont.)

Disease	Etiology	Core concepts
Myeloradiculitis	Fungal	*Cryptococcus neoformans* Some myelopathies may be secondary to vertebral osteomyelitis (*Coccidioides immitis* or *Blastomyces dermatidis*)

[a]*The diagnostic criteria for transverse myelitis include bilateral (not always symmetric) sensorimotor and autonomic spinal cord dysfunction with a clearly defined sensory level, and progression to nadir of clinical deficits between 4 h and 21 days after symptom onset. Acute myelopathy prompts the urgent need to rule out a compressive lesion. Myelitis is considered after spinal cord compression is ruled out and imaging findings are consistent with gadolinium-enhancing cord lesion along with examination of the cerebrospinal fluid. Exclusion of compressive, postradiation, neoplastic, and vascular causes is a priority. History of a recent infection is crucial to rule out the possibility of postinfectious transverse myelitis. The differential diagnosis of transverse myelitis syndrome include infectious, systemic autoimmune or inflammatory diseases, paraneoplastic causes, acquired CNS demyelinating diseases such as multiple sclerosis or neuromyelitis optica, or postinfectious or postvaccination (Frohman EM, Wingerchuck DM. Transverse myelitis. N Engl J Med 2010;**363**(6):564–572; Cho TA, Vaitkevicius H. Infectious myelopathies. Continuum Lifelong Learning Neurol 2012;**18**(6):1351–1373).*
[b]*Distinguishing spondylodiskitis among pyogenic causes, Pott's disease, and neurobrucellosis relies often on clinical and epidemiological features. However, imaging findings are often helpful to distinguish among these three conditions.*
[c]*Herpesviruses may cause of a variety of neurological manifestations including encephalitis (HSV-1, HSV-2, VZV, CMV, EBV); aseptic meningitis (VZV, HSV-2); Mollaret's meningitis (HSV-2); necrotizing retinitis (VZV, CMV); transverse myelitis (VZV, EBV, CMV); Ramsey-Hunt syndrome (VZV), Bell's palsy (HSV-1), and other neurologic syndromes.*
[d]*Verdonck K, Gonzalez E, Van Dooren S, Vandamme AM, Vanham G, Gotuzzo E. Human T-lymphotropic virus 1: recent knowledge about an ancient infection. Lancet Infect Dis 2007;(4): 266–281.*

TABLE 3.11 Infectious Causes of Neuropathies (Neuritis)[a]

Disease	Etiology	Core Concepts
Viral	*Retroviruses* Human immunodeficiency virus (HIV)	Distal symmetric polyneuropathy Multifocal neuropathy Guillain–Barre syndrome Chronic inflammatory Demyelinating Polyneuropathy (CIDP) Drug-induced polyneuropathy due to antiretroviral drugs
	HTLV-1	Tropical Spastic Paraparesis with sensorimotor, bilateral deficits affecting distal lower limbs in association with sphincter disturbances
	Herpesviruses CMV	Seen in advanced AIDS cases with usually symmetric polyneuropathy
Bacterial	*Mycobacterium leprae*	Usually present in borderline and lepromatous forms and exacerbated by leprosy reactions. In type I reactions, nerve involvement may be asymmetric and palpable due to nerve trunk thickening[b]
	Corynebacterium diphtheria	Diphteric neuropathy with bulbofacial weakness is characterized by sore throat, tonsillar exudate, and demyelinating neuropathy weeks later

TABLE 3.11 Infectious Causes of Neuropathies (Neuritis)[a] (*cont.*)

Disease	Etiology	Core Concepts
Borrelio-sis	*Borrelia burdorgferi*	Multifocal spinal root or cranial nerve involvement
		Peripheral neuropathy occurs in many patients who have meningitis. Common patterns include painful thoraco-abdominal sensory radiculitis[c]
Parasitic	*Trypanosoma cruzi*	Autonomic neuropathy with gastrointestinal involvement

[a]*Said G. Infectious neuropathies. Neurol. Clin 2007;**25**:115–137.*
[b]*White C, Franco-Paredes C. Leprosy in the 21st Century. Clin Microb Rev 2015;**28**(1):80–94. The hereditary neuropathy Dejerine-Sotas is another condition associated with palpable peripheral nerves.*
[c]*Lyme disease and syphilis may lead to sensorineural hearing loss (Rauch SD. Idiopathic sudden sensorineural hearing loss. N Engl J Med 2008;**359**(8):833–840).*

TABLE 3.12 Toxin-Mediated Nervous System Infectious Diseases[a]

Disease	Etiology	Core concepts
Botulism[b]	*Clostridium botulinum*	Different forms: • Classical (food-borne) • Infant botulism (preformed toxin is ingested) • Wound botulism (intravenous drug users or through cocaine snoring inducing sinusitis) or a wound infection with bulbar signs and descending paralysis • Hidden botulism • Inadvertent (overdose when used for aesthetic reasons)
Tetanus[c]	*Clostridium tetani*	Tetanus toxin is taken up into terminals of lower motor neurons and transported axonally to the spinal cord and/or brainstem.[d] The toxin then moves *trans*-synaptically into inhibitory nerve terminals, where vesicular release of inhibitory neurotransmitters is blocked leading to muscle ridigity and spasms manifesting as trismus, dysphagia, opistotonus and spasms of respiratory, laryngeal, and abdominal msucles leading to respiratory failure. There is also autonomic hyperactivation

[a]*Botulism develops in a stereotypical pattern with cranial nerve palsies followed by descending weakness/paralysis of the limbs and in some cases respiratory muscles paralysis. Early symptoms include blurred or double vision, dizziness, dysphagia, and slurred speech.*
[b]*Cherington M. Botulism: update and review. Semin Neurol 2004;**24**(2):155–163.*
[c]*Hassel B. Tetanus: pathophysiology, treatment, and the possibility of using botulinum toxin against tetanus-induced rigidity and spasms. Toxins 2013;(5):73–83.*
[d]*The differential diagnosis of botulism and tetanus encompasses other neuromuscular disorders including myasthenia gravias, Lambert–Eaton syndrome, Guilliain–Barre syndrome, tick paralysis, Miller–Fisher syndrome, and diphteric neuropathy.*

REFERENCES

1. Sakka L, Coll G, Chazal J. Anatomy and physiology of cerebrospinal fluid. *Eur Ann Otorhinolaryn Head Neck Dis* 2011;**128**:309–16.
2. Simon DW, Da Silva YS, Zuccoli G, Clark RSB. Acute encephalitis. *Crit Care Clin* 2013;**29**:259–77.

Chapter 4

Ocular Infections

DIAGNOSTIC APPROACH TO OCULAR INFECTIONS

Infectious Causes of Keratitis

The cornea contributes about two-thirds of the total refractive power of the human optical system.[1] Keratitis is the clinical term describing inflammation of the cornea and one of its causes includes infectious pathogens. Corneal infections often occur when there is a breach in the integrity of the corneal epithelium due to contact lenses, trauma, surgery, or existing ulcerations from other etiologies (ie, nutritional, lagophtalmos associated with leprosy). The infection occurs once the microbe enters through the epithelium into the deeper corneal stroma, which is considered an ideal medium for microbial growth.[1] In fact, infectious keratitis is a leading cause of preventable blindness worldwide and it may be due to bacteria, fungi, and protozoa (Table 4.1). However, some of the herpes viruses may also affect the cornea leading to viral keratitis. Contact lens wear is currently the most important risk factor for microbial keratitis in developed settings.[1] Among patients in whom there is a poor response to initial antibiotic treatment or those with suggestive clinical presentations, atypical pathogens such as fungal or *Acanthamoeba* must be considered.[1]

Infectious Causes of Conjunctivitis

The inner surface of the eyelid is covered by the conjunctiva (palpebral, bulbar, and limbus), which can become infected by a variety of microbes, particularly viruses and bacteria.[2] The patient's history and risk factors often provides clues to the specific diagnosis (Table 4.2). The conjunctiva produces mucus for the tear film and provides protection of the ocular surface from pathogens, and it is made up of an epithelial layer overlying the substantia propia.

Infectious Causes of Uveitis

The uvea comprises the iris, ciliary body, and choroid. The iris regulates light that reaches the retina, the ciliary body produces aqueous humor, and the choroid nourishes the retina. The uvea is the pigmented, middle layer of the eye. The

Core Concepts in Clinical Infectious Diseases (CCCID). http://dx.doi.org/10.1016/B978-0-12-804423-0.00004-4

TABLE 4.1 Infectious Etiologies of Keratitis

Category	Etiology	Core concepts
Bacterial	*Pseudomonas aeruginosa* *Serratia marcescens* *Staphylococcus aureus* *Streptococcus* spp.	Frequent association with contact lenses use and often present with rapidly progressive stromal infiltrates, suppuration and it may lead to corneal necrosis, thinning and perforation
	Less frequent (nontuberculous mycobacteria and *Nocardia*) *Treponema pallidum*	
Fungal	*Fusarium* *Candida* *Aspergillus*	More frequently occurring in tropical settings associated with agricultural trauma. It may also occur among those with long-term use of topical steroids; or contact lens wear *Fusarium* and *Aspergillus* cases described in India
Parasitic	*Acanthamoeba*	Contact lens wear
	Microsporidium	Associated with soil exposure, contact lens wear, and topical steroid use. Also may occur in patients with AIDS
	Onchocerca volvulus	Snowflake keratitis and it is an important cause of river blindness in West Africa and Latin America
Viral	Varicella–Zoster virus (VZV)	Trigeminal (V1, V2 branches) and often associated with eyelid involvement and conjunctivitis

uvea may become infected and given its location, particularly when the choroid is involved, there is an associated retinitis (chorioretinitis).[3] The classification of uveitis includes: anterior (iritis, cyclitis, iridocyclitis), intermediate (pars plana), and posterior (choroiditis, chorioretinitis, retinitis) (Table 4.3). Uveitis may involve the cornea (keratouveitis) or the sclera (sclerouveitis), and when it involves all three parts of the uvea is termed pan-uveitis. The most common infectious cause of anterior uveitis is herpes simplex infection, followed by leprosy, and Lyme's disease. Posterior uveitis is often caused by toxoplasmosis, toxocariasis, syphilis or caused by CMV. Pan-uveitis may be associated with syphilis, tuberculosis, and invasive candidiasis.[4]

TABLE 4.2 Infectious Etiologies of Conjunctivitis[a]

Category	Etiology	Core concepts
Viral	Adenovirus (causes 65–90%)	Majority of cases of acute conjunctivitis (~80%) Presents as pharyngoconjunctival fevers or epidemic keratoconjunctivitis[b] Highly contagious
Viral	Herpes virus	Comprises 1.3–4.8%
	(HSV-1/HSV-2)	Usually unilateral associated with a thin and watery discharge. Vesicular eyelid lesions are often present
	Varicella–Zoster Virus (VZV)	Associated with trigeminal herpes zoster affecting first and second branches. Eyelid involvement and conjunctivitis sometimes occur concomitantly. In some cases, keratitis and uveitis may also be present Patients with Hutchinson's sign (vesicular lesions at the tip of the nose) or eyelid involvement require expert ophthalmologic evaluation
Acute bacterial[c]	*Staphylococcus* spp. *Streptococcus pneumoniae* *Haemophilus influenzae* (In children, most often is *H. influenzae*, followed by *S. pneumoniae*, and *Moraxella catarrhalis*)	Usually lasts 7–10 days. Many cases are due to *Methicillin-Resistant S. aureus* (MRSA)
	Chlamydia trachomatis (serotypes D, E, F, G, H, I, J, K) (1.8–5.6% of cases of conjunctivitis)	Produces conjunctival hyperemia, mucopurulent discharge, and lymphoid follicle formation. It is often unilateral and have concurrent genital infection
	Chlamydia trachomatis subtypes A through C	Trachoma which is a leading cause of blindness worldwide due to late complications such as scarring of the eyelid, conjunctiva, and cornea
	Bartonella hensellae	Parinaud's oculoglandular syndrome consists of a necrotic granuloma with ulceration of the conjunctival epithelium and regional lymphadenopathy

(Continued)

TABLE 4.2 Infectious Etiologies of Conjunctivitis (*cont.*)

Category	Etiology	Core concepts
Hyperacute bacterial	*Neisseria gonorrhoeae*	Presents with severe copious purulent discharge and decreased vision. There is associated eye pain on palpation, preauricular lymphadenopathy and chemosis. High risk of corneal perforation
Chronic bacterial (>4 weeks)	*S. aureus* *Moraxella lacunata*	Red eye, purulent or mucopurulent discharge, and chemosis. Bilateral mattering of the eyelids and adherence of the eyelids, lack of itching, and no history of conjunctivitis[d]

[a]*This condition is characterized by abrupt onset of high-degree fever, pharyngitis, and bilateral conjunctivitis, periauricular lymphadenopathy.*
[b]*More severe clinical presentation is associated with watery discharge, hyperemia, chemosis, and ipsilateral periauricular lymphadenopathy. The association of conjunctivitis and lymphadenopathy occurs in approximately half of viral conjunctivitis cases and less often with bacterial causes of conjunctivitis.*
[c]*Contracted through abnormal proliferation of native conjunctival flora, oculogenital spread, contaminated fomites, and contaminated fingers.*
[d]*Other causes of conjunctivitis that need to be considered in the differential diagnosis: allergic, drug-induced, and systemic causes of conjunctivitis (Sjögren syndrome, Kawasaki disease, Stevens Johnson syndrome, and carotid cavernous fistula).*

Endophtalmitis

Infection of the vitreous or aqueous humor or both due to bacterial pathogens of fungal agents is considered as endophtalmitis,[5] and it is considered a medical emergency due to the risk of permanent vision loss. Most cases of endophtalmitis are of bacterial origin and many are exogenous due to trauma, surgery, endogenous (bacteremia or regional spread), severe keratitis, or through a glaucoma filtering bleb (Table 4.4).

Periocular Infections

This group includes infections of the eyelids, lacrimal system, and soft tissues around the orbit (Table 4.5).

TABLE 4.3 Infectious Etiologies of Uveitis (Including Retinitis)

Category[a]	Etiology	Core concepts
Viral	Rubella Chikungunya virus Zika virus Parvovirus B19	May produce anterior and posterior uveitis
	Anterior uveitis	**Hypertensive anterior uveitis**
	Varicella–Zoster virus (VZV)	Acute hypertensive anterior uveitis with granulomatous or nongranulomatous keratic precipitates (bilateral). Corneal scars maybe present and patchy or sectoral iris atrophy and vitritis. Can be seen during trigeminal zoster or associated with VZV vasculopathies
	Cytomegalovirus (CMV)	Acute anterior uveitis (Posner-Schlossman syndrome) bilateral Chronic CMV uveitis (eye discomfort and blurring)
	Herpes simplex (HSV-1 HSV-2)[b]	Presents with an injected eye and raised intraocular pressure with presence of corneal scars; unilateral HSV-1 causes keratouveitis and anterior uveitis HSV-1 and HSV-2 may cause acute retinal necrosis[c]
	Posterior uveitis	**Acute Retinal Necrosis Syndrome**
	VZV HSV-1, HSV-2 EBV, CMV	Rapid onset of pan-uveitis dominated by vitritis, vasculitis, and retinitis involving the peripheral retina (Progressive Outer Retinal Necrosis – PORN)
	Measles (subacute sclerosing panencephalitis)	Bilateral necrotizing retinitis
	CMV	CMV retinal exudates, hemorrhage, vascular sheathing, and choroidal inflammation
	West Nile virus Chikungunya	Chorioretinitis (chikungunya may also cause anterior uveitis)

(Continued)

TABLE 4.3 Infectious Etiologies of Uveitis (Including Retinitis) (*cont.*)

Category[a]	Etiology	Core concepts
Bacterial	**Anterior uveitis**	
	Neisseria meningitidis	In patients with meningococcal meningitis
	Leptospira (leptospirosis)	Weil's disease is associated with anterior uveitis10–44% of cases
	Mycobacterium leprae (leprosy)	Bilateral acute or chronic anterior uveitis
	Brucella mellitensis – Brucella abortus	Bilateral acute anterior uveitis
	T. pallidum (syphilis)	Argyll Robertson pupil is a small irregular pupil associated with anterior uveitis
	Intermediate uveitis	
	Borrelia burdorgferi (Lyme's disease)	Significant anterior segment inflammation secondary stages of Lyme's disease
	Tropheryma whippleii (Whipple's disease)	Associated with vitreous opacities and retinal-choroidal vasculitis
	Posterior uveitis	
	Bartonella hensellae	Exudative focal necrotic retinitis
Protozoan	**Posterior uveitis**	Retinitis with optic disk edema and a macular star
	Toxoplasma gondii	Exudative focal necrotic retinitis
Mycobacterial	**Posterior uveitis or Pan-uveitis** *Mycobacterium tuberculosis*	Posterior uveitis is manifested as a bilateral multifocal choroiditis with our without retinal necrosis
Fungal	*Cryptococcus neoformans*	Retrobulbar neuritis of the optic nerve produces gradual loss of vision
	Candida	May produce a chronic endophtalmitis that mimics posterior uveitis[d]
Helminthic	*Toxocara cati or Toxocara cani* (toxocariasis)	Three different clinical presentations: (1) peripheral chorioretinal granuloma; (2) posterior pole chorioretinal granuloma; and (3) pan-uveitis

[a]Many patients with anterior uveitis have inflammatory origin associated with the HLA-B27 haplotype. Other inflammatory conditions that may produce uveitis in association with other neurologic syndromes include: Behcet's disease, Sarcoidosis, Vogt–Koyanagi–Harada syndrome, Kawasaki's disease, inflammatory bowel disease, Cogan's syndrome, Wegener's granulomatosis, relapsing polychondritis, or multiple sclerosis.
[b]HSV can cause Posner-Schlossman syndrome, Fuchs uveitis syndrome, or acute iris depigmentation and pigmentary glaucoma.
[c]Acute retinal necrosis syndrome is a serious progressive ocular condition characterized by retinal necrosis, retinal vasculitis and intraocular inflammation caused by VZV, HSV-1, HSV-2, and rarely, CMV or EBV.
[d]Also, chronic infection following cataract surgery caused by Propionibacterium acnes can be associated with a a chronic pseudophakic endophtalmitis that mimics anterior uveitis.

TABLE 4.4 Etiologies of Endophtalmitis

Category[a]	Etiology	Core concepts
Acute postsurgical (cataract surgery)	*Staphylococcus epidermidis*	Other causes include *S. aureus*, streptococci, *S. pneumoniae*
Bleb-associated (surgically created for drainage of glaucoma)	*S. pneumoniae* Viridans group streptococci *H. influenzae*	
Endogenous (bacteremia or contiguous spread)	Endocarditis (*S. aureus,* viridans group streptococci) Intra-abdominal abscess (*Escherichia coli, Bacteroides*) Contiguous spread from adjacent sinusitis or orbital cellulitis	Needs to be a persistent high-grade bacteremia Invasive *Klebsiella* Syndrome (mucoid) associated with liver abscess, and other metastatic infection
Posttraumatic (exogenous)	*Bacillus cereus Staphylococcus epidermidis*	Risk factors include retained foreign body and delay in primary closure
		Less frequently: Streptococci *Klebsiella pneumoniae P. aeruginosa*
Chronic pseudophakic	*Propionibacterium acnes*	
Fungal	*Candida, Histoplasma, Coccidiodes,* and *Cryptococcus*	Disseminated disease associated with fungemia
		Candida can produce chorioretinitis or endophtalmitis/vitritis
	Aspergillus, Fusarium	Associated with cataract surgery in resource-limited settings

[a]*Durand ML. Endophtalmitis. Clin Microb Infect 2013;**19**:227–234.*

TABLE 4.5 Some Considerations About Periocular Infections

Category	Condition	Core concepts
Preseptal cellulitis (infections anterior to the orbital septum)	Etmoid sinusitis (*S. pneumoniae, S. aureus, H. influenzae*)	The lids are swollen but vision is normal, there is no afferent pupillary defect, extraocular movements are full and painless, no proptosis
Orbital cellulitis (infections posterior to the orbital septum)	Ethmoid sinusitis or sphenoid (*S. pneumoniae, S. aureus, H. influenzae*)	May lead to a subperiosteal abscess,[a] or to an orbital abscess or to cavernous sinus thrombophlebitis (suspect when contralateral signs develop)
Lacrimal system infections	Dacryocystitis	Infection of the lacrimal sac due to obstruction of the lacrimal duct (*S. aureus*, streptococci and rarely others such as *H. influenza*, Mucormycosis)
	Canaliculitis	Spontaneous or secondary to placement of punctual plugs to treat dry eyes. Associated with *Actinomyces israelii, Mycobacterium chelnei, Propionibacterium propionicum*, Eikenella, *Nocardia asteroides*
	Dacryoadenitis	Infection of the lacrimal gland (*S. aureus, P. aeruginosa*); brucellosis, and cysticercosis; viral (Epstein–Barr virus during mononucleosis); tuberculosis, Varicella–Zoster
Eyelid infections	Hordeolum	Acute infection of a sebaceous gland caused by *S. aureus*
	Chalazion	Granulomatous reaction to inspissated sebum due to and obstructed meibomian gland
	Marginal blepharitis (caused by meibomian gland dysfunction)	Diffuse inflammation of the lid margins associated with *S. aureus*
	Blepharitis/ blepharoconjunctivitis	*P. aeruginosa* *Capnotcytophaga ochracea* HSV-1
	Granulomatous blepharitis	Tuberculosis Blastomycosis

[a]*Patients with orbital cellulitis have some degree of ophtalmoplegia and proptosis. In cases of posterior orbital cellulitis (orbital apex syndrome) patients may present with severe unilateral visual loss and ophtalmoplegia but no orbital inflammation. Subperiostial abscess manifests with severe ophtalmoplegia, proptosis, deep eye pain, fever, and marked lid swelling and erythema.*

REFERENCES

1. Ong HS, Corbett MC. Corneal infections in the 21st Century. *Postgrad Med J* 2015;**91**:565–71.
2. Pleyer U, Chee SP. Current aspects on the management of viral uveitis in immunocompetent individuals. *Clin Ophtalmol* 2015;**9**:1017–28.
3. Azari AA, Barney NP. Conjunctivitis. A systematic review of diagnosis and treatment. *J Am. Med Assoc* 2013;**310**(16):1721–8.
4. Durand ML. Endophtalmitis. *Clin Microb Infect* 2013;**19**:227–34.
5. Kullberg BJ, Arendrup MC. Invasive candidiasis. *N Engl J Med* 2015;**373**(15):1445–56.

Chapter 5

Upper Airway Infections

DIAGNOSTIC APPROACH TO UPPER RESPIRATORY INFECTIONS

Acute Rhinosinusitis

Acute rhinosinusitis is the inflammation of the nasal mucosa and paranasal sinuses with obstruction of sinus ostia and impaired ciliary transport in the respiratory epithelium.[1] Viral infections are responsible for the majority of cases with superimposed bacterial infection in only 2% of cases. However, when acute bacterial infections occur, and caused by respiratory pathogens (Table 5.1), rhinosinusitis may be associated with important head and intracranial complications (Table 5.2). Oral corticosteroids combined with antibiotic may be associated with modest benefit for short-term relief of symptoms in adults with severe acute sinusitis.[2]

Acute Pharyngitis

There are many microorganisms capable of causing pharyngitis (sore throat) that could be a single disease manifestation or as part of a more generalized illness[3] (Table 5.3). There are also noninfectious causes of pharyngitis that need to be considered in the differential diagnosis of "sore throat" syndromes. Pharyngitis may be part of the common cold and this is considered one of the most common reasons for outpatient medical consultation. Acute pharyngitis in adults is associated with *Streptococcus pyogenes* in 5–9% of cases with a similar number of cases in adolescents and young adults caused by *Fusobacterium necrophorum*. Acute pharyngitis due to *S. pyogenes* is always important to suspect when an individual reports with tonsillopharyngeal exudate, tender anterior cervical lymphadenitis, and fever greater than 100.4; absence of cough and coryza (ie, Centor criteria) make the possibility of group A streptococci infection likely; particularly if this occurs during winter and early spring and when it involves school-age children. Confirmation of streptococci through antigen testing and culture is recommended. Treating group A streptococci pharyngeal infection improves symptoms, prevent further transmission, prevents rheumatic fever, and probably prevent local and systemic spread of disease.

Core Concepts in Clinical Infectious Diseases (CCCID). http://dx.doi.org/10.1016/B978-0-12-804423-0.00005-6

TABLE 5.1 Major Clinical Syndromes of the Upper Respiratory Tract

Disease	Etiologies	Core concepts
Rhinopharyngitis	*Viral* Common cold viruses (rhinoviruses, coronaviruses) Parainfluenza Influenza A and B Adenovirus Enterovirus	Fever is frequently present in children but rarely in adults. Other associated symptoms include nasal discharge that could be profuse with clear secretions that sometimes may become yellow or during the trajectory of the illness
	Bacterial *Streptococcus pneumoniae* *Haemophilus influenza* *Staphylococcus aureus* *Moraxella catarrhalis* *Streptococcus* spp. Anaerobes	Less common than viral
Pharyngitis	Infectious Non-infectious	Bacterial, viral, chlamydial, mycoplasmal, or candida Drug induced, Still's disease, Kawasaki's disease, gastroesophageal reflux disease
Pertussis	*Bordetella pertussis*	Three clinical phases including the following: 1. Catarrhal (7–10 days with predominant upper respiratory symptoms) 2. Paroxysmal (1–6 weeks with episodic cough) 3. Convalescent (7–10 Days) of gradual recovery
Otitis media	Bacterial *S. pneumoniae* *H. influenza* *S. aureus* *M. catarrhalis* *Streptococcus* spp.	Complications of acute otitis media include mastoiditis, brain abscess of the temporal lobe, lateral venous sinus thrombosis, and otitis media with effusion
	Treponema pallidum during secondary syphilis	Otitis malignant externa is associated invasion of temporal bone via cartilage of external auditory canal *S. aureus* or *Pseudomonas aeruginosa* in patients with diabetes mellitus or severely immunocompromised (ie, HIV/AIDS)

TABLE 5.1 Major Clinical Syndromes of the Upper Respiratory Tract (*cont.*)

Disease	Etiologies	Core concepts
Epiglottitis	Bacterial or viral *H. influenza* *S. aureus*	Rapid progression to high fever, toxic appearance, drooling, and respiratory distress with no coughing May occur in children 2–5 years of age but cases are also seen in adolescents and young adults. "Thumb sign" which corresponds to the large swollen epiglottis is present on lateral neck radiograph Management priority is establishing an airway and antibiotic coverage including vancomycin and usually a third generation cephalosporin to cover *H. influenzae* or other respiratory pathogens

Among adolescents and young adults (usually 15–18 years of age) presenting with acute pharyngitis, fever, tender cervical lymphadenopathy and a scarlatiniform rash and whose evaluation is negative for *S. pyogenes* or infectious mononucleosis, infection due to *Archanobacterium haemolyticum* should be suspected.

TABLE 5.2 Complications of Bacterial Rhinosinusitis

Anatomic location	Complications
Maxillary	Possibly brain abscesses through emissary veins
Frontal	Potts puffy tumor associated with osteomyelitis and subperiostal abscess of the frontal bone, brain abscess (frontal lobe), epidural abscess, subdural empyema, meningitis (trauma leading to CSF leakage)
Sphenoid	Posterior orbital abscess, cavernous sinus thrombosis, venous sinus thrombosis, meningitis
Ethmoid	Preseptal cellulitis (see chapter: Ocular Infections), subperiostial abscess, orbital abscess, cavernous sinus thrombosis, meningitis

TABLE 5.3 Differential Diagnosis of Acute Pharyngitis[a]

Etiologies	Syndrome	Core concepts
Bacterial	*S. pyogenes*	Can cause pharyngitis, tonsillitis, scarlet fever, rheumatic fever, glomerulonephritis, reactive arthritis, PANDAS[b] Patients usually have sore throat, cervical adenopathy but there is no rhinorrea, coryza, or cough
	Streptococcus dysgalactiae subspecies *equisimilis* (Group C streptococci)	Pharyngitis and tonsillitis Glomerulonephritis (most commonly when it causes skin and soft tissue infections)
	Neisseria gonorrhoeae	Can cause pharyngitis and it is sexually acquired and maybe associated with disseminated gonococcal infection
	A. haemolyticum	Pharyngitis and scarlatiniform rash
	Corynebacterium diphtheriae	Severe pharyngitis with peripheral neuropathy and myocarditis
Viral[c]	Human immunodeficiency virus (HIV)	Acute retroviral syndrome associated with HIV
	Epstein-Barr virus	Infectious mononucleosis
	Cytomegalovirus	Infectious mononucleosis
	Human Herpes Virus-6 (HHV-6)	Mononucleosis-like illness with pharyngitis
	Adenovirus types 3, 4, 7, 14 and 21	Pharyngoconjunctival fever
	Herpes simplex types 1 and 2	Stomatitis, pharyngitis
	Coxsackievirus A types 2, 4, 5, 6, 8, and 10	Herpangina
Chlamydial	*Chlamydia pneumoniae*	Pneumonia, bronchitis, pharyngitis
Mycoplasmal	*Mycoplasma pneumoniae*	Pneumonia, bronchitis, pharyngitis
Inflammatory[d]	Adult onset Still's disease	Pharyngitis (although, there is some evidence that soreness maybe due to laryngeal cartilage inflammation)
	Kawasaki's disease	Mucocutaneous syndrome that may involve the pharynx
Parasitic	*Toxoplasma gondii*	Mononucleosis-like illness that can include pharyngitis

TABLE 5.3 Differential Diagnosis of Acute Pharyngitis[a] (*cont.*)

Etiologies	Syndrome	Core concepts
Fungal	*Candida albicans*	Oral and esophageal candidiasis
Drug induced	Angiotension converting enzyme inhibitors Erythema multiforme with mucosal involvement	
Miscellaneous noninfec-tious[e]	Smoking Snoring Endotracheal intubation Gastroesophagel reflux Air pollution	

[a]*Bisno AL. Acute pharyngitis. N Engl J Med 2001;**344**(3):205–211.*
[b]*Pediatric autoimmune neuropsychiatric disorders associated with streptococcal infection.*
[c]*Influenza A and B may have include some component of pharyngitis given its involvement of many segments of the upper and lower respiratory epithelium; similarly parainfluenza 1–4 may cause symptoms consistent with common cold and croup that could involve sore throat.*
[d]*Renner B, Mueller CA, Shephard A. Environmental and non-infectious factors in the aetiology of pharyngitis (sore throat). Inflamm Res 2012;61:1041–1052.*
[e]*Other processes that can cause pharyngitis include Epiglottitis (infectious) can cause pharyngitis if associated with severe inflammation) or Ludwig's angina or retropharyngeal abscess.*

Chronic Cough Syndrome

The syndrome of chronic cough (>12 weeks) is also an important reason for infectious disease consultation and it can be caused by chronic smoking, post nasal drip due to chronic bacterial sinusitis, gastroesophageal reflux, anatomic abnormalities of the respiratory tract, drug-induced angiotensin-converting enzyme inhibitors (ACE), pertussis,[4] asthma, and chronic interstitial lung disease. Diagnostic workup of chronic should consider this differential diagnosis.

Bronchorrhea

Bronchorrhea is defined as water sputum production of over 100 mL per day and sometimes it can be confused as a chronic cough syndrome. The most important considerations in the differential diagnosis include primary lung malignancies including bronchioloalveolar carcinoma since it involves some glandular component that produces excess mucous. Bronchorrhea can also be associated with lung metastases form adenocarcinomas of the colon, pancreas, or other glands. Nonmalignant conditions include endobronchial tuberculosis, and asthma. Patients with ruptured pulmonary echinococcosis (hydatid disease) into a bronchus may also present with bronchorrhea and often report a salty taste associated with expectoration.

TABLE 5.4 Odontogenic Infectious Syndromes

Syndrome/disease	Core concepts
Noma (cancrum oris)[a]	It is a polymicrobial infection that destroys the hard and soft tissues of the mouth and may involve the nose and other parts of the face Its an ulcerative disease of extreme poverty that occurs concomitantly or immediately after a debilitating illness such as measles, malaria, severe enterocolitis, tuberculosis, or necrotizing ulcerative gingivitis Most important pathogens are *F. necrophorum* and *Prevotella intermedia* and due to its effect on nutrition, its associated with stunt growth, malnutrition, and often death
Lemierre's syndrome[b]	Septic thrombophlebitis of the jugular vein that sometimes is associated with odontogenic infection with secondary seeding of the jugular vein. Patients often present with cavitary lung lesions due to multiple septic emboli to the lung or pleural effusions/empyemas
Submandibular abscesses and Ludwig's angina	Usually arise from the spread of periapical abscess of the mandibular molars, most typically from the second or third molar Periapical abscess involving the first molar initially infect the sublingual space, whereas infections originating from the 2nd or 3rd molar infect the submylohyoid space and this infection pushes the tongue against the epiglottis Ludwig's angina experience a rapid spreading woody inflammation of the submandibular area that can lead to insidious or rapidly progressive asphyxiation if left untreated
Brain abscess[c]	Connection through the valveless emissary veins leading to brain abscesses usually temporal or parietal lobes (see chapter: Central Nervous System Infections)

[a]*Enwonwu CO. Noma – the ulcer of extreme poverty. N Engl J Med 2006;**354**;(3):221–224.*
[b]*Reynolds SC, Chow AW. Life-threatening infections of the peripharyngeal and deep fascial spaces of the head and neck. Infect Dis Clin. N Am 2007;**21**:557–576.*
[c]*Brouwer MC, Tunkel AR, McKhann II GM, van den Beek D. Brain abscess. N Engl J Med 2014;**371**(5):447–456; Darouiche RO. Spinal epidural abscess. N Engl J Med 2006;**355**(19):2012–2020.*

Septic Thrombophlebitis of the Internal Jugular Vein (Lemierre's Syndrome)

Lemierre's syndrome is septic thrombophlebitis of the internal jugular vein.[1] *F. necrophorum* is the most common pathogen associated with this disease, and previously it was recognized as postanginal sepsis due to *S. pyogenes* pharyngitis.[5] It most often steams from ear, nose, and throat infections that spread into the vasculature that drains through the jugular vein.[6] Septic embolization to the

TABLE 5.5 Necrotizing Syndromes of the Nose and Nasopharynx[a]

Infections and inflammatory conditions involving the nasal mucosa and cartilaginous portion	Saddle nose deformity	Syphilis Leprosy Granulomatosis with polyangiitis Relapsing polychondritis Midline granulmoma
	Vestibulitis with our without abscess	Methicillin Resistant *S. aureus* (MRSA) usually community-associated and highly-associated with smoking Less frequently caused by *S. pneumoniae* or *Haemophilus* spp.
	Parasitic	Mucocutaneous leishmaniasis due to *L. braziliensis*
	Mycobacterial	*Mycobacterium leprae*
	Rhinoscleroma[b]	*Klebisella rhinoscleromatis* produces a chronic granlumoatous disease of the nose of other parts of the respiratory system including palate, and larynx
	Noma (cancrum oris)[c]	Polymicrobial including oral anaerobes
	Fungal	Paracoccidiodomycosis, blastomycosis, histoplasmosis, and coccidiodomycosis
	Granulomatous	Sarcoidosis
	Malignancy	Squamous cell carcinoma, basal cell carcinoma, lymphoma
	Miscellaneous	Chronic and frequent snoring of cocaine

[a]*Reynolds SC, Chow AW. Life-threatening infections of the peripharyngeal and deep fascial spaces of the head and neck. Infect Dis Clin N Am 2007;**21**:557–576.*
[b]*Gaafar HA, Gaafar AH, Nour YA. Rhinoscleroma: An updated experience through the last 10 years. Acta Octo-Laryngologica 2011;**131**:440–446.*
[c]*Enwonwu CO. Noma-The ulcer of extreme poverty. N Engl J Med 2006;**354**;(3):221–224.*

lungs is often considered part of this syndrome.[6] These cases occurred in an era before antibiotics, when this illness had a mortality rate of 90%. After the introduction of antibiotics in the 1950s, Lemierre's syndrome vanished for several decades. Interestingly, in the past two decades, there have been at least 400 cases reported in the literature through case studies and many cases are caused invasive community-acquired methicillin resistant *S. aureus* MRSA.[6]

The differential diagnosis of selected odontogenic infectious syndromes and necrotizing infectious processes of the nose are discussed in Table 5.4 and Table 5.5, respectively.

REFERENCES

1. Chow AW, Benninger MS, Brook I, Brozek JL, Goldstein EJC, Hicks LA, et al. IDSA clinical practice guideline for acute bacterial rhinosinusitis in children and adults. *Clin Infect Dis* 2012;**54**(8):1041–5.
2. Venekamp RP, Thompson MJ, Rovers MM. Systemic corticosteroid therapy for acute sinusitis. *JAMA* 2015;**313**(12):1258–9.
3. Bisno AL. Acute pharyngitis. *N Engl J Med* 2001;**344**(3):205–11.
4. Hewlett EL, Edwards KM. Pertussis – not just for kids. *N Engl J Med* 2005;**352**(12):1215–22.
5. Kizhner V, et al. Methicillin-resistant *Staphylococcus aureus* bacteraemia associated with Lemierre's syndrome: case report and literature review. *J Laryngol Otol* 2013;**127.7**:721–3.
6. Chanin JM, Marcos LA, Thompson BM, et al. Methicillin-Resistant *Staphylococcus aureus* USA 300 clone as a cause of Lemierre's syndrome. *J Clin Microb* 2011;**49**(5):2063–6.

Chapter 6

Lower Airway Infections

DIAGNOSTIC APPROACH TO LOWER RESPIRATORY INFECTIONS

Most causes of pneumonia are caused by common bacterial respiratory pathogens.[1] In the clinical expression of pneumonia syndromes, there is a complex interaction among viral, bacterial, and host factors. By combining the host characteristics with environmental influences and exposures there is a wide spectrum of potential infectious causes of pneumonia. Microaspiration of bacterial colonizers of the oropharynx and nasopharynx is the most frequently pathophysiologic mechanism underlying pneumonia. Macroaspiration (large volume) of gastric contents into the airway is associated with the syndrome of "aspiration pneumonitis." However, in some cases, there is a synergistic damage induced by viral and bacterial coinfection: for example, coinfection due to respiratory syncytial virus (RSV) and bacterial; or influenza and *Streptococcus pneumoniae;* or influenza and *Staphylococcus aureus* coinfection.[2] Influenza viral infection contributes to respiratory epithelial cell dysfunction of protein synthesis and apoptosis.

Among patients presenting with pneumonia from the community, it is important to distinguish it from hospital-acquired pneumonia. The rationale for distinguishing between these two clinical syndromes relies on the type of oral bacterial colonizers or dwellers. Since the mechanism of acquiring pneumonia is microaspiration colonization with frequent bacterial oral colonizers acquired in the community is radically different than those bacterial dwellers of the nasopharynx or oropharynx acquired in the hospital. Bacterial pathogens associated with community-acquired pneumonia include *S. pneumoniae*, *Haemophilus influenzae*, and *Moraxella catarrhalis*; and atypical pathogens such as *Legionella pneumophila, Mycoplasma pneumoniae, and Chlamydia pneumoniae.*

The pathophysiologic mechanism underlying hospital-acquired pneumonia including ventilator-associated pneumonia is microaspiration of oropharyngeal, upper gastrointestinal, or subglottic contents (Table 6.1). In the health-care setting, microaspiration phenomena including Gram-negative bacilli often with a multidrug pattern of antimicrobial susceptibility are capable of escaping the

Core Concepts in Clinical Infectious Diseases (CCCID). http://dx.doi.org/10.1016/B978-0-12-804423-0.00006-8

TABLE 6.1 Clinical Syndromes Associated With Aspiration[a]

Clinical syndrome	Core concepts
Bland aspiration without clinical consequences	Aspiration of blood due to epistaxis or hematemesis Aspiration of enteral feedings Postesophagogastroduodenoscopy (20% of cases)
Chemical pneumonitis[b]	Associated with anesthesia (Mendelson's syndrome) Consists of a spectrum of disease that starts with aspiration of liquid gastric contents recovers within 36 h with no clear permanent sequelae to transient hypoxemia to acute respiratory distress syndrome (ARDS)
Anaerobic pleuropneumonia	*Subacute presentation* with cough productive of purulent, often foul-smelling sputum, and cavitary pneumonia with an associated empyema Patients usually have a history of loss of consciousness days to weeks earlier
Community-acquired pneumonia and health-care-associated pneumonia	Microaspiration of oropharyngeal or nasopharyngeal content (CAP) Microaspiration of gastrointestinal, oropharyngeal, nasopharyngeal, or subglottic contents (ventilator associated pneumonia)[c]
Aspiration pneumonia	*Acute lung infection* developing after a large-volume aspiration of oropharyngeal or upper gastrointestinal contents with a high enough pH to not cause chemical pneumonitis In some cases, infection due to nonvirulent, predominantly anaerobic microorganisms is secondary to a large bacterial inoculum (higher bacterial content is associated with poor dental hygiene); or when there are more than 3 predominant types of anaerobic pathogens Represent 10–15% cases of hospital acquired pneumonias

[a]*DiBardino DM, Wunderink RG. Aspiration pneumonia: a review of modern trends. J Crit Care 2015;**30**:40–48.*
[b]*Pneumonitis refers to parenchymal inflammation of the lung (interstitial and alveolar) caused by noninfectious factors compared to pneumonia which is caused by infectious agents. In both conditions, there is an inflammatory response inside the lungs*
[c]*Pneumonia is a major cause of death associated with cerebrovascular accidents associated with a reduced subset of lymphocytes (invariant natural T cells) that causes a rapid depression of the cellular immune response that takes place as a response to the stroke (Meisel C, Meisel A. Suppressing immunosuppression after stroke. N Engl J Med 2011;**365**(22):2134–2136).*

biocidal action of antimicrobials, collectively representing major medical challenges in the pathogenesis and management of health-care-associated infections (ie, *Klebsiella pneumoniae, Pseudomonas aeruginosa, Enterobacter* spp., *Serratia* spp., *Escherichia coli*, and Methicillin-resistant *Staphylococcus aureus*).[3] Multiple acronyms such have dubbed this group of pathogens: SPACE (*Serratia, Providencia, Acinetobacter, Citrobacter,* and *Enterobacter*) or ESKAPE (*Enterococcus faecium, Staphyloccus aureus, K. pneumoniae, Acinetobacer baumannii, P. aeruginosa, and Enterobacter* spp.). Risk factors for acquiring health-care associated pathogens includes: (1) intravenous therapy, wound care, or intravenous chemotherapy within the prior 30 days; (2) nursing home resident or long-term care facility; (3) hospitalization in the prior 3 months; and (4) hemodialysis.

The clinical syndromes of bronchitis, including trachebronchitis, laryngotracheitis are noted in Table 6.2. Pneumonia is a major cause of illness and death worldwide.

Cavitary Lung Disease

Pulmonary parenchymal cavities are caused by tissue necrosis that leads to the exclusion of a portion of the pulmonary parenchyma via the bronchial tree. In general, the differential diagnosis of pneumonitis with cavitations includes infectious and noninfectious inflammatory etiologies (Table 6.3). The infectious causes includes bacteria community-associated *methicillin* resistant *Staphylococcus aureus, Actinomyces or nocardia asteroides, Rhodococcus equi, P. aeruginosa,* melioidosis, polymicrobial necrotizing pneumonias or lung abscesses; mycobacteria including *Mycobacterium tuberculosis* or nontuberculous mycobacteria such as *Mycobacterium kansasiii, Mycobacterium avium-intracellulare* and others, fungi *Aspergillus fumigatus, Histoplasma capsulatum, Cryptococcus neoformans or Cryptococcus gatti, Blastomyces dermatitidis, Coccidiodes immitis, Penicillium* and others; and parasites *Paragonimus westermani*, or cystic echinococcosis. Other infectious causes include septic emboli to the lung (right-sided endocarditis, infected vascular catheter or Lemierre's syndrome).[4–11]

Among the noninfectious inflammatory or autoimmune causes of cavitary lung disease, the most salient etiologies include autoimmune diseases such as granulomatosis with polyangitis, eosinophilic granulomatosis and polyangiitis, rheumatoid arthritis, sarcoidosis, ankylosing spondylitis.[5] Additionally, pulmonary contusion and pulmonary infarction may lead to cavitary disease. Neoplasias such as bronchogenic carcinomas (most frequently squamous cell carcinoma) or metastatic neoplasms to the lung may develop into cavities; or else a bronchogenic carcinoma may lead to postobstructive pneumonia with secondary cavitation.[4,12] Thick wall cavities compared to thinner ones, tend to be associated with malignancies (Table 6.3).[4,5,12]

TABLE 6.2 Clinical Spectrum and Differential Diagnosis of Lower Respiratory Tract Infections

Category	Etiology	Core concepts
Laryngotracheitis	Most cases of laryngotracheitis are caused by parainfluenza virus and influenza	Patients start with symptoms of a viral upper respiratory infection (coryza, rhinorrhea, cough, and fever) followed by inspiratory stridor, a barking cough and hoarseness
Acute bronchitis	Inflammation of the bronchial tree	Viral or bacterial causing inflammation of the bronchial wall with increased secretions, cough, fever, pharyngitis, and malaise
	Smoking and gastric acid reflux are also important bronchial irritants	Most common viral pathogens include rhinovirus, influenza, respiratory syncytial virus (RSV)
Bronchiolitis	Most frequently cause by RSV or parainfluenza	Most common cause of hospital admissions due to respiratory illnesses in infants (<1 year of age)
	Influenza may also be associated with bronchiolitis	
Pneumonia	Community-acquired pneumonia	Microaspiration of oropharyngeal, or nasopharyngeal flora causing alveolar inflammation with community-acquired pathogens (typical and atypical pathogens)
	Hospital-acquired pneumonia	Microaspiration of oropharyngeal, nasopharyngeal, gastrointestinal, or subglottic contents (Gram-negative resistant pathogens or MRSA)
	Aspiration pneumonias	Macroaspiration of oropharyngeal, nasopharyngeal, gastrointestinal with development of acute pneumonia (15% of aspiration pneumonias are caused by macroaspiration)
Chronic bronchitis	Related to smoking Viral infection may exacerbate episodes of chronic bronchitis	Daily cough and sputum production for at least 3 months for 2 years or longer
Empyema	Thoracic empyema is the accumulation of pus in the pleural fluid through direct contamination of the pleural space, spread of contiguous infection from peripheral lung infections	Associated with pneumonia in more than 60% of cases and of bacterial origin: S. pneumoniae, anaerobes, viridans group streptococci, Gram-negative rods, Candida spp. Other causes include: Esophageal rupture/tear (boerhaave syndrome) Thoracic or abdominal surgery Tuberculosis Trauma

TABLE 6.3 Etiologies of Cavitary Pulmonary Disease[a]

Category	Differential diagnosis
Infectious	*Bacterial* Necrotizing pneumonias (ie, *Staphylococcus aureus, S. pneumoniae, K. pneumoniae, P. aeruginosa*) Lung abscesses (frequently polymicrobial from oral bacterial flora) Septic pulmonary emboli (ie, *Staphylococcus aureus*) Lemierre's syndrome (*Fusobacterium necrophorum or Staphylococcus aureus*) Actinomycosis Melioidosis *Rhodococcus* *Parasitic* Paragonimiasis Echinococcosis *Mycobacterial* *M. tuberculosis* Non-tuberculous mycobacteria (ie, *M. kansasii, Mycobacterium avium-intracellulare, Mycobacterium abscessus*) *Fungal* Aspergillosis Histoplasmosis Blastomycosis Coccidiodomycosis Cryptococcosis *Penicillium* *Pneumocystis jiroveci* Paracoccidiodomycosis Zygomicosis
Inflammatory	Granulomatosis and polyangiitis Rheumatoid arthritis Ankylosing spondylitis Sarcoidosis Microscopic polyangiitis Eosinophilic granulomatosis and polyangiitis Granulomatosis and polyangiitis
Neoplastic	Squamous cell carcinoma of the lung Lymphoma Kaposi's sarcoma
Miscellaneous	Pulmonary infarction Fat embolism Langerhan's cell histiocytosis Cryptogenic organizing pneumonia (formerly bronchiolitis obliterans organizing pneumonia or BOOP)

[a]*Franco-Paredes C. Aerobic actinomycetes that masquerade as pulmonary tuberculosis. Bol Med Hosp Infant Mex 2014;71(1):36–40.*

Acute Pulmonary Infiltrates, Fever and Respiratory Failure Syndromes

The association of pulmonary infiltrates, fever, and associated respiratory failure pose a major challenge to clinicians, particularly when patients present with no previously significant risk factors. Obtaining a detailed clinical history is crucial including recent travel, exposures, medications, vectors (mosquitoes, ticks, or others), and existing medical conditions (ie, diabetes, transplantation, immunodeficiencies, and others). The differential diagnosis of subacute or chronic illness characterized by episodic fever, alveolar/interstitial pulmonary infiltrates, and respiratory failure is depicted in Table 6.4. The differential

TABLE 6.4 Differential Diagnosis of Acute Febrile Illness, Pulmonary Infiltrates (Alveolar and/or Interstitial) and Respiratory Failure[a]

Category	Etiology and description
Inflammatory	Acute interstitial pneumonitis (Hamman–Rich syndrome)
Cardiac	Exacerbation of heart failure sometimes with concomitant respiratory infection (i.e., influenza)
Aspiration pneumonia (different than anaerobic pleuropneumonia)	Aspiration pneumonia there is an infectious process presenting acutely Anaerobic Pleuropneumonia is associated with a subacute course
Diffuse alveolar hemorrhage	ANCA-associated vasculitis (granulomatosis and polyangiitis, eosinophilic granulomatosis and polyangiitis, microscopic polyangiitis) Antiglomerular basement antibodies (Goodpasture's syndrome is caused by antibodies against the first non-collagenous domain of the alpha-3 chain of collagen type IV in the lung and the kidney) Antiphospholipid syndrome Systemic lupus erythematosus Behcet's syndrome Henoch–Schönlein purpura
Drug induced	Diffuse alveolar damage (aspirin, bleomycin, methotrexate cyclophosphamide) Alveolar hemorrhage (anticoagulants, phenytoin, amphotericin B, cyclophosphamide, nitrofurantoin) Nonspecific interstitial pneumonia (amiodarone, nitrofurantoin, sufasalazine) Cryptogenic organizing pneumonia (BOOP or caused by amiodarone, nitrofurantoin, methotrexate, carbamazepine) Eosinophilic Pneumonia (nitrofurantoin, amiodarone, bleomycin, phenytoin, hydrochlorothiazide, penicillamine)

TABLE 6.4 Differential Diagnosis of Acute Febrile Illness, Pulmonary Infiltrates (Alveolar and/or Interstitial) and Respiratory Failure[a] (*cont.*)

Category	Etiology and description
Hypersensitivity pneumonitis	Extrinsic allergic alveolitis (environmental exposure and there is no peripheral eosinophilia)
Pulmonary alveolar proteinosis	Associated with anti-GM-CSF antibodies leading to pulmonary alveolar proteinosis. The presence of anti-GM-CSF has also been associated as a risk factor for *Cryptococcus gattii* infections in otherwise immunocompetent individuals
Acute eosinophilic pneumonia	No peripheral eosinophilia, bronchoalveolar lavage with more than 25% of eosinophils
Fungal	Cryptococcosis Histoplasmosis Blastomycosis Paracoccidiodoymycosis Coccidiodomycosis *Penicillium marneffei* *Pneumocytis jiroveci*
Tickborne	*Francisella tularensis* (Tularemia) *Rickettsia* (Rocky Mountain spotted fever) *Ehrlichia chaffeensis* or *Ehrlichia ewingii* (Human granulocytic ehrlichiosis) *Babesia microti* *Borrelia burdorgferi*
Viral	Influenza Epstein–Barr virus Herpes simplex virus (rare but reported among otherwise immunocompetent individuals)
Unusual bacterial	*Francisella tularensis* (Tularemia) *Coxiella burnetti* (Q fever) *Yersinia pestis* (Plague)

Anti-GM-CSF (antigranulocyte macrophage colony stimulating factor).
[a]*Other than community-acquired pneumonia (typical and atypical respiratory pathogens) and hospital acquired pneumonia.*

diagnosis of interstitial pulmonary infiltrates to consider during infections diseases consultations is listed in Table 6.5.

Tuberculosis-Like Pneumonias

Acid-fastness is a physical property of some microorganisms by resisting decolorization by acids during staining procedure that is clinically useful. There are other respiratory microorganisms other than *M. tuberculosis* and the nontuberculous mycobacteria that share the ability of staining acid fast

TABLE 6.5 Differential Diagnosis of Selected Interstitial Lung Diseases

Categories	Associated conditions
Autoimmune	Systemic lupus erythematosus Rheumatoid arthritis Scleroderma Dermatomyositis
Sarcoidosis	Disease may manifest with bilateral hilar adenopathy such as in the Löfgren's syndrome or diffuse bilateral infiltrates and sometimes with cavitary disease due to extensive lung injury (Stage IV)
Eosinophilic granuloma	Presents usually in females, smokers and sometimes there is a history of spontaneous pneumothorax
Lymphangioleiomyomatosis	Occurs in premenopausal women with pulmonary infiltrates associated with infiltration of smooth muscle cells and sometimes mimicking emphysema
Vasculitis	Granulomatosis with polyangiitis Lymphomatoid granulomatosis Bronchogenic granulomatosis Eosinophilic granulomatosis and polyangiitis (also called Churg–Strauss syndrome—sometimes unmasked when using leukotrienes for the treatment of severe asthma)
Eosinophilic pneumonias	Acute and chronic alveolar injury of unknown etiology
Pulmonary alveolar proteinosis	Associated with hematologic malignancies, idiopathic, toxins but often associated with the presence of antigranulocyte-macrophage colony-stimulating factor (anti-GM-CSF)
Idiopathic pulmonary hemosiderosis	Sometimes associated with systemic lupus erythematosus but most cases are of idiopathic origin
Goodpasture's syndrome	Antibasement membrane antibodies causing pulmonary hemorrhage and hematuria
Idiopathic Pneumonia Syndrome	Posthematopoietic stem cell transplantation: idiopathic pneumonia syndrome[a]

[a]This is an acute lung dysfunction of noninfectious etiology and considered a complication following hematopoietic stem cell transplantation with widespread alveolar injury, absence of infection, and no cardiac or renal etiology (Panoskaltsis-Mortar A, Griese M, Madtes DK, Belperio JA, Hadda IY, Folz RJ. An official American Thoracic Society research statement: noninfectious lung injury after hematopoietic stem cell transplantation: idiopathic pneumonia syndrome. Am J Respir Crit Care Med 2011;**183**:1262–1279).

including *Nocardia* spp., *Rhodococcus* spp., *Tsukamurella* sp., and *Legionella micdadei*. Therefore, clinicians should consider this group of pathogens in the differential diagnosis of tuberculosis like-pneumonias.[13]

Indeed, the *Actinomycetales* group of bacterial pathogens includes phylogenetically diverse but morphologically similar aerobic and anaerobic actinomycetes such as *Actinomyces, Rothia, Nocardia, Williamsia, Gordonia, Tsukamurella*, and *Rhodococcus*. This group of pathogens can cause lung infections associated with cavitary lesions and a clinical syndrome consistent with productive cough for many weeks, hemoptysis, fever, night sweats, weight loss and malaise that resembles pulmonary tuberculosis.[1] These organisms may not only mimic pulmonary tuberculosis by their clinical and radiographic features but they may also appear as acid-fast bacilli in respiratory specimens. *Rhodococcus* spp. infection affects immunocompromised individuals and pulmonary disease is present in about 80% of cases with the most common radiographic findings being cavitary pneumonia located in the upper lobes.

Bronchiectasis

Bronchiectasis are abnormal anatomic dilatations of bronchioles and bronchi that manifest with productive cough and repeated episodes of respiratory infections, hemoptysis, and disabling dyspnea.[14] Bronchiectasis represents an acquired disorder that was considered at some point the direct result of recurrent respiratory infections during childhood. Nonetheless, with the availability of an armamentarium of broad-spectrum antimicrobials, effective treatment of pulmonary tuberculosis along with routine immunization programs in childhood, the rate of bronchiectasis in the population has decreased. Bronchiectasis can present in either of two forms: as a local or focal obstructive process of a lobe or segment of an affected lobe and a diffuse process involving both lungs (Table 6.6). When the disease is bilateral diffuse, it tends to be associated with sinopulmonary diseases such as sinusitis and asthma.

The most important risk factor for the development of bronchiectasis is necrotizing pneumonias due to *Stapylococcus aureus, P. aeruginosa*, and likely due to recurrent aspiration pneumonitis when is caused by large volume aspiration of gastric residues. Other risk factors include, infections due to non-tuberculous mycobacteria such as *Mycobacterium avium-intracellulare*, cystic fibrosis, dyskinetic cilia syndrome, and allergic bronchopulmonary aspergillosis (ABPA). Patients experience with large amount of mucopurulent thick sputum, or sometimes dry cough. The most common etiologies of bronchiectasis are noted in Table 6.6. Preventing further infections is the only potential mechanism for breaking the vicious cycle of bronchial transmural infection and inflammation.[7] Often, patients require long-term antibiotic suppression with rotating antibiotics with the goal of preventing repeated.

Pulmonary Alveolar Proteinosis

Granulocyte-macrophage colony-stimulating factor (GM-CSF) regulates innate immune cells, including macrophages, neutrophils, and dendritic cells. It is a central effector for Th1-type cytokine production. Anti-GM-CSF autoantibodies

TABLE 6.6 Clinical Spectrum and Differential Diagnosis of Bronchiectasis[a]

Categories	Etiologies	Core concepts
Autoimmune	Rheumatoid arthritis Systemic lupus Erythematosus Relapsing polychondritis Scleroderma Sjögren syndrome	Sometimes also associated with chronic pleural effusions
Postinfectious	Bacterial Mycobacterial Fungal Viral	*Pseudomonas* spp. *H. influenzae* *Staphylococcus aureus* *Mycobacterium avium-intracellulare* *M. tuberculosis* *Aspergillus* spp. Adenovirus, Measles Influenza HIV
Immunodeficiency	Common variable immunodeficiency Secondary hypogammaglobulinemia Chronic lymphocytic leukemia Chemotherapy-induced	Sinopulmonary infections leading frequently to bronchiectasis *Mycobacterium avium-intracellulare* causing a vicious cycle of bronchiectasis ensuing a predisposition for further MAC or other non-tuberculous mycobacteria
Toxin induced	Foreign body Heroin overdose Chlorine exposure	
Inflammatory	Allergic bronchopulmonary aspergillosis (ABPA) Inflammatory bowel disease Young's disease	Central bronchiectasis A hypersensitivity reaction of *Aspergillus* spp. colonizing the airways in association with asthma Secondary ciliary dyskinesis

TABLE 6.6 Clinical Spectrum and Differential Diagnosis of Bronchiectasis[a] (cont.)

Categories	Etiologies	Core concepts
Congenital	Primary ciliary dyskinesis	Kartagener's syndrome (bronchiectasis, sinusitis, and situs inversus or partial lateralizing abnormality)
	Cystic fibrosis	Associated with *Burkhordelia cepacia, Pseudomonas* spp.
	Tracheobronchomegaly	(Mounier–Kuhn syndrome)
	Cartilage deficiency	(Williams–Campbell syndrome)
	Pulmonary sequestration	
	Marfan's syndrome	
	Alpha$_1$-antitrypsin deficiency	

[a]*Barker AF. Bronchiectasis.* N Engl J Med *2002;**346**(18):1383–1391.*

have been identified as a pathogenic factor in the occurrence of pulmonary alveolar proteinosis (PAP). In this condition, macrophage dysfunction associated with the presence of anti-GM-CSF antibodies produces pulmonary infiltrates secondary to decreased clearance of phospholipoproteinaceous material leading to their alveolar accumulation impairing gas exchange and dyspnea. There are hematological disorders, immunodeficiencies, chronic infections, and toxic factors that trigger PAP. There is a crazy paving associated with interlobular septal thickening with superimposed ground glass opacities in computed tomography imaging. Patients with anti-GM-CSF autoantibodies are also at increased risk of *C. gattii* central nervous system infection.[15] The most common conditions that need to be considered in the differential diagnosis of PAP include: (1) bronchioloalveolar carcinoma; (2) *Pneumocystis jiroveci* pneumonia (PCP); (3) diffuse alveolar hemorrhage, and (4) alveolar sarcoidosis. Confirmation of the diagnosis of PAP is by demonstration amorphous, acellular, eosinophilic periodic acid-Schiff-positive material.[16]

REFERENCES

1. Chertow DS, Memoli MJ. Bacterial coinfection in influenza. *JAMA* 2013;**309**(3):275–82.
2. Hunt DP, Muse VV, Pitman MB. Case 12-2013: an 18-year-old woman with pulmonary infiltrates and respiratory failure. *N Engl J Med* 2013;**368**(16):1537–45.
3. Pendleton JN, Gorman SP, Gilmore BF. Clinical relevance of ESKAPE pathogens. *Expert Rev Anti Infect Ther* 2013;**11**(3):297–308.

4. Gallant JE, Ko AH. Cavitary pulmonary lesions in patients infected with human immunodeficiency virus. *Clin Infect Dis* 1996;**22**(4):671–82.
5. Gadkowski LB, Stout JE. Cavitary pulmonary disease. *Clin Microb Rev* 2008;**21**(2):305–33.
6. Hidron AI, Low CE, Honig EG, et al. Emergence of community-acquired methicillin-resistant *Staphylococcus aureus* strain USA 300 as a cause of necrotizing community-onset pneumonia. *Lancet Infect Dis* 2009;**9**(6):384–92.
7. Yamschikov AV, Schuetz A, Lyon MG. *Rhodococcus equi* infection. *Lancet Infect Dis* 2010;**10**:350–8.
8. Wallace Jr RJ, Glassroth J, Griffith DE, et al. Diagnosis and treatment of disease caused by nontuberculous mycobacteria. *Am J Resp Crit Care Med* 1997;**156**:S1–S25.
9. Griffith DE, Girard WM, Wallace Jr RJ. Clinical features of pulmonary disease caused by rapidly growing mycobacteria. An analysis of 154 patients. *Am Rev Respir Dis* 1993;**147**(5):1271–8.
10. Blumberg HM, Leonard MK, Jasmer RM. Update on the treatment of tuberculosis and latent tuberculosis infection. *JAMA* 2005;**293**(22):2776–84.
11. Weinstock DM, Brown AE. *Rhodococcus equi*: an emerging pathogen. *Clin Infect Dis* 2002;**34**:1379–85.
12. Franco-Paredes C. Aerobic actinomycetes that masquerade as pulmonary tuberculosis. *Bol Med Hosp Infant Mex* 2014;**71**(1):36–40.
13. Savini V, Fazii P, Favaro M, Astolfi D, Polilli E, Pompilio A, et al. Tuberculos-like pneumonias by the aerobic actinomycetes *Rhodoccocus, Tsukamurella,* and *Gordonia*. *Microb Infect* 2012;**14**:401–10.
14. Barker AF. Bronchiectasis. *N Engl J Med* 2002;**346**(18):1383–91.
15. Saijo T, Chen J, Chen SCA, Rosen LB, Jin Y, Sorrell TC, et al. Anti-granulocyte macrophage colony-stimulating factor autoantibodies are a risk factor for central nervous infection by *Cryptococcus gattii* in otherwise immunocompetent patients. *mBio* 2014;**5**(2):1–8.
16. Patel SM, Sekiguchi H, Reynolds JP, Krowka MJ. Pulmonary alveolar proteinosis. *Can Resp J* 2012;**19**(4):243–53.

Chapter 7

Neck and Thoracic Infections

DIAGNOSTIC APPROACH TO THORACIC AND NECK INFECTIONS

Endarteritis/Endovascular Infection

Endovascular infections are defined as bloodstream infections in which continuous viable bacteria are detected in blood cultures (bacteremia) despite the institution of adequate antimicrobial therapy.[1,2] The target cell of endovascular infection is the endothelial cell of the lining of the great vessels. Staphylococci avidly adhere to endothelial cells and bind through adhesion interactions triggering the phagocytosis of the bacterium by endothelial cells. Once intracellularly, small-colony variants formed allowing the bacterium to develop persistent infection and shelter from the immune system attack with the eventual risk of recurrent returning to the bloodstream to thrive by obtaining nutrition by iron obtained through producing hemolysin that releases iron from erythrocytes during bacteremia. The invasion of endothelial cells by *Staphylococcus aureus* triggers the expression of tissue factor that initiates a cascade of events that promotes the development of vegetations in damaged or undamaged endocardium of valvular surfaces.[3]

Although *S. aureus* may use vascular endothelial cells to thrive and produce a true endovascular infection, this term refers to infection of the wall of large vessels belonging to the systemic, pulmonary, or venous system and often resulting in aneurysms, pseudoaneurysms, or even arteriovenous fistulae.[1] Common bacterial pathogens that cause endovascular infections include *Salmonella*, *Abiotrophia*, and *Granulicatella* species. In this context, infection of the endocardium/cardiac valves as part of endocarditis should be considered within the spectrum of endovascular infections[2] (see chapter: Bloodstream Infections). In summary, although continuous or persistent bacteremia despite institution of therapy is a feature of endovascular infections, this group of infections imply infection of the wall of a large vessel (endarteritis) or the endocardium (endocarditis).[1,3]

The complications of *S. aureus* bacteremia include: (1) prosthetic device infection, (2) Henoch–Schonlein purpura, (3) Waterhouse–Friderichsen syndrome, and (4) metastatic infection (vertebral osteomyelitis, spleen abscess, epidural abscess, purulent mediastinitis, purulent pericarditis, and others).

Core Concepts in Clinical Infectious Diseases (CCCID). http://dx.doi.org/10.1016/B978-0-12-804423-0.00007-X

Infective Endocarditis

Infective endocarditis is the result of infection of the endocardium (internal lining of the heart) and of the heart valves.[4–6] With the myriad of today's health-care associated factors that predispose to infection, the epidemiology of infective endocarditis has become quite complex. Despite improved medical and surgical advances, the clinical outcomes of infective endocarditis have not been affected. It continues to be major form of life-threatening infection along with sepsis, pneumonia, and intraabdominal abscess. The clinical expression of infective endocarditis depends on the host response, the virulence of the organism, and predisposing risk factors. There is also a spectrum of disease associated with culture negative endocarditis. In this clinical syndrome, there are different mechanisms that translate into no detectable bacterial growth in blood cultures. The most relevant causes of culture negative endocarditis include: (1) recent or present use of antibiotics; (2) infection due to fastidious organisms such as the HACEK group, *Coxiella burnetti, Bartonella hensellae,* or brucellosis; and (3) nonbacterial thrombotic (marantic or cachectic) endocarditis (Fig. 7.1).

Currently, the most common and most important cause of infectious endocarditis is caused by *S. aureus*. Combined, staphylococci and streptococci account for approximately 80% of case of infective endocarditis, with *S. aureus* currently considered the most common pathogen (Table 7.1).[4–6]. Complications of the central nervous system are considered the most severe extracardiac manifestations of infective endocarditis. Neurologic complications are associated with infection caused by *S. aureus* and with vegetations that are large, mobile, or in the mitral position.[6] Indications for surgery include heart failure, uncontrolled infection, and prevention of embolic events.[6,7] Indications for antibiotic prophylaxis to undergo invasive dental procedures among individuals with prosthetic heart valves include having a history of infective endocarditis, or unrepaired cyanotic congenital heart disease (Table 7.2).[5]

Nonbacterial Thrombotic Endocarditis

Infectious endocarditis is a genuine primary suppurative infection of the endocardium and cardiac valves, whereas nonbacterial thrombotic endocarditis (NBTE) is a noninflammatory expression of a hypercoagulable state, which is most notably a paraneoplastic syndrome.[7–9] Cachectic (marantic or terminal type) endocarditis can be divided in two groups: one in which embolism is clinically evident, and a second one in which embolism is occult. Marantic endocarditis is not prone to become secondarily infected suggesting that a preexisting thrombus plays a minor role, if any, in the pathogenesis of infective endocarditis.[8]

Heyde's Syndrome

This syndrome is associated with submucosal angiodysplasia causing gastrointestinal bleeding in patients with calcific aortic stenosis, which then may be

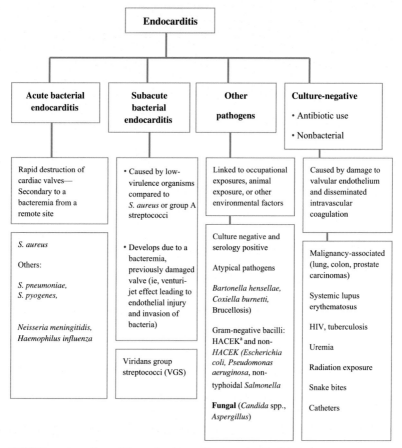

FIGURE 7.1   **Diagnostic approach to differential diagnosis of endocarditis.**

a predisposing risk factor for aortic valve endocarditis. Heyde's syndrome is a form of type IIA von Willebrand's syndrome, an acquired deficiency of high-molecular-weight von Willebrand factor multimers.[10] Acquired deficiency of von Willebrand factor is a rare and has been described in patients with monoclonal gammopathy of undetermined significance, multiple myeloma and it has been associated with gastrointestinal dysplasia and bleeding. Among patients with aortic-valve stenosis, loss of high-molecular weight multimers is associated with abnormalities in platelet adhesion and aggregation in vitro. The cause of the deficiency of high-molecular weight von Willebrand factor multimers in Heyde's syndrome is a consequence of shear stress through a stenotic aortic valve altering the conformation of high-molecular-weight von Willebrand factor and exposing sites that can be cleaved by the plasma protease ADAMTS13.

TABLE 7.1 Categories of Infective Endocarditis[a]

Category	Description	Core concepts
Native valve	*S. aureus* *Streptococcus pyogenes* *Streptococcus agalactiae* *Streptococcus pneumoniae* Viridans group streptococci	Acute bacterial endocarditis with rapid valve destruction Stigmata include conjunctival petechiae, splinter hemorrhages, or embolic disease Cause subacute bacterial endocarditis (SBE) given its lower virulence and it is often associated with immunologic-induced stigmata such as Osler's nodes and Janeway lesions
Prosthetic valve	*Staphylococcus* coagulase negative	Early infections arises within 60 days or surgery and late infections after 60 days
Nosocomial	*S. aureus* Enterococci *Staphylococcus* coagulase negative	Risk factors include: hemodialysis, catheters, or surgical procedures
Intravenous drug users[b]	*S. aureus* *Pseudomonas aeruginosa* Fungal (*Candida* spp.)	Intravenous drug use, but cases also associated with subcutaneous (skin popping) of speed (combinations of cocaine and heroine)

[a]The diagnosis of infective endocarditis relies on the modified Duke criteria which comprises microbiologic, echocardiographic, and clinical-laboratory criteria (Baddour LM, Wilson WR, Bayer AS, Fowler VG, Tleyjeh IM, Rybak MJ, et al. Infective endocarditis in adults: diagnosis, antimicrobial therapy, and management of complications. A scientific statement for healthcare professionals from the American Heart Association. Circulation 2015;**132**:1435.
[b]Lowy FD, Gordon RJ. Bacterial infections in drug users. N Engl J Med 2005;**353**(18):1945–1954.

Consequently, the high-weight multimers are reduced in size and hemostatically less competent. Since von Willebrand factor is essential for the well-known role of platelets in maintaining vascular integrity independent of their essential role in homeostasis, this combination of factors has been responsible for explaining the onset of angiodysplasias.[10]

Myocarditis

Cardiac insufficiency evolving into cardiogenic shock and death is the most severe complication in the short term or dilated cardiomyopathy with chronic heart failure is the most concerning long-term sequelae associated with acute myocarditis. Acute myocarditis is most often caused by viral infections, but

TABLE 7.2 Infection Syndromes in Illicit Drug Users

Category	Description/core concepts
Sexually transmitted Viral Bacterial	HIV, CMV, HTLV-1 *Chlamydia trachomatis, Neisseria gonorrhoeae,* *Treponema pallidum*
IVDU Parasitic Viral Bloodstream bacterial	*Leishmania donovani* (visceral leishmaniasis) in patients with HIV/AIDS and IVDU[a] HIV, hepatitis B, Hepatitis C *S. aureus,* group A, B, G streptococci *P. aeruginosa* (it may cause sternoclavicular septic arthritis)
Bacterial skin and soft tissue infections	*S. aureus* Viridans group streptococci HACEK Group A, B, C, G streptococci *P. aeruginosa, Klebsiella, Escherichia coli, Serratia* *marscescens* *Aeromonas* spp *Mycobacterium tuberculosis*
Toxin mediated	Botulism (black tar heroin use) Tetanus Toxic Shock Syndrome due to either *S. aureus* or *S. pyogenes*
Respiratory bacterial	Tuberculosis Community-acquired pneumonia Opportunistic pulmonary infections (HIV-related) Tuberculosis, *Nocardia, P. aeruginosa,* *Rhodococcus equi* Aspiration pneumonitis

IVDU, Intravenous drug use.
[a]Cruz I, Morales MA, Noguer I, Rodriguez A, Alvar J. Leishmania *in discarded syringes from intravenous drug users.* Lancet 2002;**359**(9312):1124–1125.

there is also a growing recognition of parasitic infections to the burden of disease associated with myocardial infections[11] (Table 7.3). In particular, Chagas cardiomyopathy remains as a major public health challenge in Latin America and in countries with an increasing number of immigrant populations from endemic settings.[12]

Another form of cardiac injury induced by parasitic infections include parasite-induced hypereosinophilia which has been associated with tropical endomyocardial fibrosis.[13] The clinical presentations of tropical endomyocardial fibrosis are similar to those of the idiopathic hypereosinophilic syndrome when it involves the heart.[13] Circulating eosinophils many undergo characteristic changes that have been associated with cellular activation and eosinophil-induced tissue damage. This results in endomyocardial fibrosis, which may be manifested

TABLE 7.3 Differential Diagnosis of Infectious and Noninfectious Inflammatory Causes of Myocarditis[a]

Category	Etiology	Disease/Syndrome
Parasitic	Chagas disease(American trypanosomiasis) *Trypanosoma cruzi*[b]	Chagas heart disease (CHD) is the most common etiology of cardiomyopathy in Latin America, and a major cause of cardiovascular death among middle-aged individuals in endemic areas. It manifests as three major syndromes that often coexist in the same patient: arrhythmic, heart failure, and thromboembolism In CHD, arrhythmias are very common and of different types, frequently associated, and may cause palpitations, dizziness, syncope, and sudden cardiac death (SCD) Frequent, complex PVCs, including couplets and runs of NSVT, are a common finding on 24-h Heart failure is often a late manifestation of CHD. It is usually biventricular with predominance of left-sided failure at initial stages and of right-sided failure at more advanced disease. Systemic and pulmonary embolisms arising from mural thrombi in the cardiac chambers are quite frequent. Sudden cardiac death is the main cause of death in patients with CHD, accounting for nearly two-thirds of all deaths, followed by refractory heart failure, and thromboembolism
	Human African trypanosomiasis (caused by *Trypanosoma brucei rhodesiense*)	Myocarditis, with occasional pancarditis may occasionally develop during the hemolymphatic stage, leading to arrhythmias and heart failure with *T. b rhodesiense* infection. The pathophysiology of cardiac involvement in African trypanosomiasis is secondary to endarteritis and fibrosis caused by perivascular infiltration by trypanosomes and lymphocytes. Diagnosis is made by visualization of the trypanosomes from chancre fluid, lymph node aspirates, blood, or cerebrospinal fluid
	Toxoplasmosis Myocarditis, pericardial effusion, constrictive pericarditis, arrhythmias and congestive heart failure have been described in patients infected with *Toxoplasma gondii*	*T. gondii* associated myocarditis can also occur in transplant patients either due to a reactivation or to *de novo* infection from a seropositive donor to a seronegative recipient

	Trichinellosis (caused by *Trichinella spiralis* and has a worldwide distribution; humans become infected when eating undercooked contaminated meat)	Trichinellosis associated myocarditis is not caused by the direct larval invasion of the myocardium with encystation but likely induced by an eosinophilic-enriched inflammatory response resulting in eosinophilic myocarditis similar to the pathogenic process associated to tropical endomyocardial fibrosis. In addition, pericardial effusions have also been reported during *T. spiralis* infection. The clinical suspicion of trichinellosis is based on the epidemiology associated with the typical clinical presentation and the presence of eosinophilia; confirmation is based on serology and muscle biopsy
		The tropism of *T. spiralis* for striated muscle may lead to involvement of the myocardium in 21–75% of infected patients. Complications such cardiac arrhythmias are considered the most common cause of death associated to trichinellosis
Viral	Lymphocytic myocarditis most likely of viral origin (viral genomes present in 35% of cases)	Heart failure with dilated left ventricle but no atrioventricular blocks or arrhythmias
		Associated with good prognosis
	Nonspecific myocarditis with inflammatory cells most likely of viral origin (viral genomes present in 25–35% of cases)	Heart failure with dilated left ventricle without new ventricular arrhythmias or high degree atrioventricular block
		Prognosis of this clinical syndrome depends of functional class ejection fraction

(Continued)

TABLE 7.3 Differential Diagnosis of Infectious and Noninfectious Inflammatory Causes of Myocarditis[a] (cont.)

Category	Etiology	Disease/Syndrome
Inflammatory	Necrotizing eosinophilic myocarditis Giant-cell myocarditis	Manifesting as an acute myocardial infarction-like syndrome with normal coronary arteries. Patients with lymphocytic infiltration on myocardial biopsy have a good prognosis
	Acute lymphocytic myocarditis (or less frequently giant-cell myocarditis or necrotizing eosinophilic) Acute lymphocytic, necrotizing eosinophilic or giant cell myocarditis	Heart failure with normal size left ventricle or dilated left ventricle and hemodynamic instability. Often requires inotropic or mechanical circulatory myocarditis Overall prognosis is good for fulminant lymphocytic myocarditis Heat failure with dilated left ventricle and high-degree atrioventricular block and new ventricular arrhythmias Poor prognosis and it is considered an indication for heart transplantation
Inflammatory with eosino-philia	Hypersensitivity or hypersensitivity myocarditis	Heart failure with peripheral eosinophilia. Requires high-dose corticosteroids and carries a poor prognosis
Granulomatous	Sarcoidosis Idiopathic granulomatous myocarditis Chagas Disease, Lyme disease	Heart failure with dilated left ventricle, new ventricular arrhythmias, high degree block and lack of response to usual care within 2 weeks of symptom onset

[a]In patients with high suspicion of chronic CD or in those with a compatible clinical syndrome, because parasitemia is scarce, the presence of IgG antibodies against T cruzi antigens needs to be detected by at least two different serological methods (usually enzyme-linked immunosorbent assay, indirect immunofluorescence, or indirect haemagglutination) to confirm the etiological diagnosis.
[b]Franco-Paredes C, Rouphael N, Mendez J, Folch E, Rodriguez-Morales AJ, Santos JI, et al. Cardiac manifestations of parasitic infections. Clin Cardiol 2007;**30**:218–222.

clinically as restrictive cardiomyopathy. This process leads to endomyocardial fibrosis, mural thrombus formation, arrhythmias, and pericarditis with effusion in some cases. Filariae and schistosomiasis are the most frequently nematodes inducing chronic eosinophilia with consequent endomyocardial fibrosis.[13]

Mediastinitis

Mediastinitis is defined as an inflammation of connective tissue that involves mediastinal structures and involving interpleural spaces.[14–16] There are noninfectious inflammatory causes and infectious causes. Most cases are associated with cardiac surgery, usually post-CABG (coronary artery bypass grafting).[16] Other clinically relevant etiologies include esophageal perforation (Boerhaave's syndrome), tracheobronchial perforation/fistula, mediastinal extension of pulmonary infections, or the extension of peripharyngeal and deep fascial spaces of the head and neck, particularly from the retropharyngeal space through the danger zone. Specific etiologies of descending mediastinitis include odontogenic infections, retropharyngeal abscess, peritonsillar abscess, cervical lymphadenitis, sternoclavicular septic arthritis, external trauma, and parotitis and thyroidits. Management of mediastinitis often involves surgical or percutaneous drainage, along with antimicrobial therapy and supportive care. Boerhaave's syndrome has been associated with pertussis and influenza infections.

The Postpericardiotomy Syndrome

The postpericardiotomy is a complication following cardiac surgery and manifesting as an inflammatory pleuropericardial syndrome affecting about 15–20% of patients.[17] The overall prognosis is good but constrictive syndrome may occur in a minority of patients. The inflammatory reaction occurs due to pericardial or pleural trauma, or both and manifests with fever, severe and debilitating dry cough, pleuritic chest pain and elevation of inflammatory markers. Pericardial bleeding is considered a trigger for the syndrome within the spectrum of postcardiac injury inflammatory syndromes. The postpericardiotomy syndrome is considered with the spectrum of disease of Dressler's syndrome, which is considered an immunologically mediated pericarditis induced from a myocardial infection and thus also termed postmyocardial infarction syndrome or postcardiac injury syndrome. Management of the syndrome requires thoracocentesis and/or pericardiocenthesis depending on the degree of involvement of the pleural and pericardial spaces along with the use of antiinflammatory therapies (corticosteroids and nonsteroidal antiinflammatory drugs). Colchicine has shown to be of limited value in the treatment of this syndrome, but it may have a value in preventing this condition.[17] The postpericardiotomy syndrome must be clinically distinguished from acute mediastinitis. A key distinguishing factor is that despite the severity of symptoms associated with the postpericardiotomy syndrome and overlap of signs and symptoms with mediastinitis, patients with infectious mediastinitis progress rapidly to severe sepsis and septic shock.

Pericarditis

Inflammation of the pericardium may be the result of infectious, inflammatory (including Autoinflammatory), postcardiac injury syndromes, neoplastic processes, and other miscellaneous conditions[18–20] (Table 7.4).

TABLE 7.4 Differential Diagnosis of Pericarditis[a]

Category	Description	Core concepts
Infectious	Tuberculosis	Concomitant disease often, particularly during acute disseminated tuberculosis (primary progressive tuberculosis)
	Bacterial suppurative (purulent)	Requires early surgical intervention
	Viral	Echo, Coxsackie, Epstein–Barr virus, HIV, parvovirus B19
	Borrelial	Lyme's disease
	Rickettsial	Q fever (*Coxiella burnetii*)
	Fungal	Histoplasmosis, blastomycosis, *Aspergillus* spp., *Candida* spp., *Cryptococcus neoformans*
Metastatic	Squamous cell carcinoma	
	Lung	
	Breast	
	Lymphoma	
Immune-mediated injury	Dressler syndrome	Postmyocardial infarction
	Postperiocardiotomy syndrome	Postcardiac surgery. Important to distinguish clinically from infectious mediastinitis. Responds to antiinflammatory therapy and drainage of pleural/pericardial fluid if indicated
	Autoimmune	Systemic lupus erythematosus. Rheumatoid arthritis. Inflammatory bowel disease. Sjögrens syndrome. Scleroderma
	Autoinflammatory	Familial mediterranean fever, tumor-necrosis factor-associated periodic syndrome
	Systemic vasculitis	Eosinophilic granulomatosis with polyangiitis. Takayasu's. Behcet's disease

TABLE 7.4 Differential Diagnosis of Pericarditis[a] (*cont.*)

Category	Description	Core concepts
Constrictive pericarditis	Postinfectious Neoplastic Postsurgical/trauma Renal failure Idiopathic	Tuberculosis Fungal (histoplasmosis) Metastatic disease to pericardium Mediastinal irradiation Cardiac trauma or surgery
HIV associated	Infectious etiologies	*S. aureus, M. avium-intracellulare, R. equi,* Cytomegalovirus, *Cryptococcus neoformans, Histoplasma capsulatum,* Epstein–Barr, HHV-8 (body cavity lymphoma)
Neoplastic	Primary neoplastic	Pericardial mesothelioma
Metabolic	Uremia, hypothyroidism	
Drug-related	Lupus-like syndrome Hypersensitivity Direct injury	Procainamide, hydralazine, isoniazid, phenytoin Beta-lactam antibiotics Antineoplastic drugs (doxorubicin, cyclophosphamide)
Traumatic/ iatrogenic	Esophageal perforation Postperiocardiotomy syndrome	

[a]*Imazio M, Gaita F, LeWinter M. Evaluation and treatment of pericarditis. A systematic review. JAMA 2015;**314**(14):1498–1506.*

Neck Infections Associated Syndromes

Peritonsillar, parapharyngeal and retropharyngeal abscess are considered deep neck infections originated from contiguous spread of a surrounding infectious process (Table 7.5). These processes share some overlapping clinical manifestations and if not diagnosed early they are life-threatening.[21–27]

Peritonsillar or Quinsy abscesses is a usually unilateral collection of pus outside the tonsillar capsule located in the region of the upper pole of the tonsil and involving the soft palate.[23–25] The infection usually starts in the intratonsillar fossa and extends around the tonsil. Quinsy abscess affects more often children than adults. Retropharyngeal abscesses occur mostly in early childhood and it is caused by the spread of an oral cavity infection to the retropharyngeal lymph nodes. Infection of the retropharyngeal, parapharyngeal, and lateral space needs early clinical diagnosis and prompt surgical intervention along with effective antimicrobial therapy. Within the clinical spectrum of neck infections, salivary gland non-infectious inflammatory and infectious processes, particularly of the parotid gland, consist of a broad differential diagnosis.[28] Suppurative thyroiditis caused by Streptococcus pneumonia, S. aureus or by anaerobes need to also be considered (Table 7.6).

TABLE 7.5 Life Threatening Infections of the Head and Neck

Location	Core concepts
Submandibular space	Tooth infection determines site of infection (infections of the apex of the 2nd and 3rd molar are associated with submylohyoid space, whereas infections of the 1st molar lead to submandibular infection) Source of infection includes odontogenic, fractures, lacerations, or foreign bodies Submandibular swelling but no trismus
Lateral pharyngeal space	*Anterior compartment* Patients present with sepsis and dysphagia, neck pain, and/ or trismus. Requires surgery due to purulent nature and its original infectious source is tonsillitis *Posterior compartment* This infections do not cause trismus but may lead to septic jugular phlebitis May involve carotid sheath and result in Horner's syndrome, 9th to 12th cranial nerve palsies, or arterial rupture
Retropharyngeal space	Infection usually originates in deep cervical lymph nodes or from trauma. Infections entering the retropharyngeal and danger spaces may lead to mediastinitis. Prevertebral space infections are generally due to seeding via the hematogenous route, similar to epidural abscess or vertebral osteodiscitis

TABLE 7.6 Differential Diagnosis for Unilateral Parotid Enlargement[a]

Category	Core concepts
Acute bacterial suppurative parotitis[b]	*S. aureus* is the most commonly identified etiology followed by anaerobic bacteria (*Prevotella* and *Porphyromonas* spp., *Fusobacterium* spp., and *Peptostreptococcus* spp. Streptococci including *S. pneumoniae* and Gram-negative bacilli have also been reported *Burkholderia pseudomallei* (melioidosis) usually manifests as pneumonia, and multiple abscesses including parotid infection.[c] Affects persons who are in regular contact with soil and water. Diabetes mellitus is a risk factor for severe disease, followed by alcohol abuse, chronic renal disease, thalassemia, cancer therapy, and use of corticosteroids. In Australia, there is a high rate of prostatitis and neurologic involvement Treatment of parotid abscess requires surgical drainage along with specific antimicrobial therapy
Infectious nonsuppurative	Viral (HIV, influenza, coxsackievirus, Epstein–Barr virus, lymphocytic coriomeningitis virus (LCM), parainfluenza, herpes simplex virus, CMV Mycobacterial (*Mycobacterium tuberculosis* and *Mycobacterium avium-intracellulare*)

TABLE 7.6 Differential Diagnosis for Unilateral Parotid Enlargement[a] *(cont.)*

Category	Core concepts
	Fungal (*Candida albicans, Cryptococcus neoformans, Coccidioides immitis, H. capsulatum*) Treponemal: *T. pallidum*
Autoimmune/in-flammatory	Mikulicz syndrome[d] Sjögren's syndrome IgG-4-related syndrome Kimura's disease (eosinophilic lymphofolliculosis is characterized by deep subcutaneous masses involving primarily the head and neck region Associated regional lymphadenopathy and salivary gland involvement with eosinophilic infiltration and elevated IgE levels Diffuse infiltrative lymphocytosis syndrome (DILS—in HIV infection some individuals may develop bilateral but sometimes unilateral cystic disease of the parotid gland) Sarcoidosis (Heerfordt–Waldenström syndrome)
Neoplastic	Lymphoma Leukemia Primary non-Hodgkin's lymphoma (MALToma) Benign lymphoepithelial lesions Pleomorphic adenoma Angiolipoma, parotid oncocytoma, Warthin tumor (most likely bilateral) Parotid hemangioma Facial nerve neurofibroma Malignant (acinus cell carcinoma, adenoid cystic carcinoma, mucoepidermoid carcinoma, parotid adenocarcinoma, rhabdomyosarcoma, rhabdomyosarcoma) Metastatic disease (squamous cell carcinoma, malignant melanoma, thyroid carcinoma Congenital (first brachial cleft cyst)
Viral	Mumps HIV
Miscellaneous	Pneumoparotid Sialolithiasis associated usually with hyperparathyroidism Sialosis

[a]*Tang CG, Nuyen BA, Puligandia B, Rasgon B. The coccidioidomycosis conundrum: a rare parotid mass. Perm J 2014;**18**(2):86–88; Brook I. Acute bacterial suppurative parotitis: microbiology and management. J Craniofac Surg 2003;**14**(1):37–40.*
[b]*When pus is obtained by milking the Stensen duct by the health-care provider.*
[c]*Melioidosis is the third most common cause of death from infectious disease in northeast Thailand, exceeded only by tuberculosis and HIV infection and it is also frequent in Australia. Cases of melioidosis occur in other Asian countries, and some countries in Latin America, the Caribbean, and some areas in Africa but likely this infectious agent has a worldwide distribution (Wiersinga WJ, Currie BJ, Peacock SJ. Melioidosis. N Engl J Med 2012;**367**(11):1035–1044).*
[d]*Mikulicz syndrome is a chronic condition characterized by the abnormal enlargement of glands in the head and neck, including those near the ears (parotids) and those around the eyes (lacrimal) and mouth (salivary). The tonsils and other glands in the soft tissue of the face and neck may also be involved. Although the disorder is almost always described as benign, it always occurs in association with another underlying disorder such as tuberculosis, leukemia, syphilis, Hodgkin's disease, lymphosarcoma, Sjögren syndrome, or lupus (SLE). People who have Mikulicz syndrome are at heightened risk for developing lymphomas.*

TABLE 7.7 Infections of the Chest Wall

Category	Etiology	Core concepts
Empyema necessitans (also termed empyema necessitatits)	Extension of empyema from pleural cavity to the surrounding structures to the chest wall or to other surrounding structures (mediastinum, pericardium, etc.)	*M. tuberculosis* Actinomyces spp. (thoracic actinomycosis) *S. aureus* (USA 300 MRSA) *Mucormycosis* Fusobacterium spp. Blastomyces dermatitis Aspergillus spp.
Costochondritis (Tietze syndrome)	Rare inflammatory disorder of unknown cause	Multiple microtrauma to the chest wall is probably a contributing factor Some cases associated with psoriatic arthritis
Dermatomal herpes zoster	Varicella–Zoster virus	May present single dermatome or multiple one sided dermatomes can be involved
Pleurodynia ("The devil's grip," Bornholm's disease)	Coxsackie B3 Echovirus Coxsackie A	Usually presents in epidemic settings with severe spasmodic pain in the chest or upper abdomen associated with fever
Mondor's disease	Superficial thrombophlebitis of the breast and/or thoracic wall	Benign condition
Necrotizing skin and soft tissue infections	Necrotizing fasciitis type I – polymicrobial or type 2 (*S. pyogenes* or *Aeromonas hydrophila*)	Associated with placement of tube thoracostomy for empyema or postsurgical chest procedures Spontaneous or associated with minor trauma Requires aggressive debridement due to high case fatality rate
Parasitic infections	Gnathostomiasis (*Gnathostoma spinigerium*)	Migration of larval parasite through chest wall produces a painful subcutaneous swelling associated with peripheral eosinophilia. A small area of ecchymosis is sometimes identified
	Cutaneous larva currens	Caused by entry of *Strongyloides stercolaris* through chest wall causing a creeping eruption. Sometimes it may be caused by cutaneous larva migrans due to *Ancylostoma brasiliensis*

Infections of the Chest Wall

Some infectious diseases may affect the chest wall and producing mild benign conditions to life-threatening necrotizing infections (Table 7.7).

REFERENCES

1. Olsen EGJ. Endovascular infections. *Postrad Med J* 1989;**65**:127–8.
2. Mohajer MA, Darouiche RO. Sepsis syndrome, bloodstream infections, and device-related infections. *Med Clin North Am* 2012;**96**:1203–23.
3. Lowy FD. *Staphylococcus aureus* infections. *N Engl J Med* 1998;**339**(8):521–32.
4. Hoen B, Duval X. Infective endocarditis. *N Engl. J Med* 2013;**368**:1425–33.
5. Baddour LM, Wilson WR, Bayer AS, Fowler VG, Tleyjeh IM, Rybak MJ, et al. Infective endocarditis in adults: diagnosis, antimicrobial therapy, and management of complications. A scientific statement for healthcare professionals from the American Heart Association. *Circulation* 2015;**132**:1435.
6. Moreillon P, Que YA. Infective endocarditis. *Lancet* 2004;**363**:139–46.
7. Lopes JA, Ross RS, Fishbein MC. Nonbacterial thrombotic endocarditis: a review. *Am Heart J* 1987;**113**(3):773–84.
8. Steiner I. Nonbacterial thrombotic versus infective endocarditis: a necropsy study of 320 cases. *Cardiovasc Pathol* 1995;**4**(3):207–9.
9. Johnson JA, Everett BM, Katz JT, Loscalzo J. Painful purple toes. *N Engl J Med* 2010;**362**:67–73.
10. Loscalzo J. From clinical observation to mechanism – Heyde's syndrome. *N Engl J Med* 2012;**367**(20):1954–6.
11. Cooper LT. Myocarditis. *N Engl J Med* 2009;**360**(15):1526–38.
12. Franco-Paredes C, Bottazzi ME, Hotez PJ. The unfinished public health agenda of Chagas disease in the era of globalization. *PLoS Neglect Trop Dis* 2009;**3**(7):e470.
13. Franco-Paredes C, Rouphael N, Mendez J, Folch E, Rodriguez-Morales AJ, Santos JI, et al. Cardiac manifestations of parasitic diseases Part 3: pericardial and miscellaneous cardiopulmonary manifestations. *Clin Cardiol* 2007;**30**:277–80.
14. Inaco Cirino LM, Melhem Elias F, de Almeida JLJ. Descending mediastinitis: a review. *Sao Paulo Med J* 2006;**124**(5):285–90.
15. El Oakley RM, Wright JE. Postoperative mediastinitis: classification and management. *Ann Thorac Surg* 1996;**61**:1030–6.
16. Risnes I, Abdelnoor M, Almdahl SM, Svennevig JL. Mediastinitis after coronary artery bypass grafting risk factors and long-term survival. *Ann Thorac Surg* 2010;**89**:1502–10.
17. Imazio M. The post-pericardiotomy syndrome. *Curr Opin Pulm Med* 2012;**18**:366–74.
18. LeWinter MM. Acute pericarditis. *N Engl J Med* 371;**25**:2410–2416.
19. Imazio M, Gaita F, LeWinter M. Evaluation and treatment of pericarditis. A systematic review. *JAMA* 2015;**314**(14):1498–506.
20. Hoit BD. Management of effusive and constrictive pericardial disease. *Circulation* 2002;**105**:2939–42.
21. Reynolds SC, Chow AW. Life-threatening infections of the peripharyngeal and deep fascial spaces of the head and neck. *Infect Dis Clin North Am* 2007;**21**:557–76.
22. Brook I. Current management of upper respiratory tract and head and neck infections. *Eur Arch Otorhinolaryngol* 2009;**266**:315–23.
23. Brook I. Microbiology and management of peritonsillar, retropharyngeal, and parapharyngeal abscesses. *J Oral Maxillofac Surg* 2004;**62**:1545–50.

24. Caruso G, Passali FM, Salerni L, Molinaro G, Messina M. Head and neck mycobacterial infections in pediatric patients. *Int J Pediatr Otorrhinolaryngol* 2009;**73S**:S38–41.

25. Schubert AD, Hotz MA, Caversaccio MD, Arnold A. Septic thrombosis of the internal jugular vein: Lemierre's Syndrome revisited. *Laryngoscope* 2015;**125**(4):863–8.

26. Brook I. Current management of upper respiratory tract and head and neck infections. *Eur Arch Otorrhinolaryngol* 2009;**266**:315–23.

27. Brook I. Microbiology and principles of antimicrobial therapy for head and neck infections. *Infect Dis Clin North Am* 2007;**21**:355–91.

28. Tang CG, Nuyen BA, Puligandia B, Rasgon B. The coccidiodomycosis conundrum: a rare parotid mass. *Perm J* 2014;**18**(2):86–8.

Chapter 8

Abdominal/Pelvic Infections

DIAGNOSTIC APPROACH TO ABDOMINAL AND PELVIC INFECTIONS

The most common signs and symptoms associated with abdominal and pelvic infectious syndromes include acute pain, chronic pain associated with fever, jaundice, nausea, vomiting, dysphagia, and diarrhea or constipation. Acute and chronic forms of pancreatitis are an important source of morbidity and mortality; and associated with a high hospitalization rate. The two most important causes of acute pancreatitis include gallstone obstruction of the biliary tract and alcohol consumption.[1] Nonetheless, there are also a few pathogens that directly invade the pancreas such as Coxsackievirus or even *Mycobacterium tuberculosis* or drug-induced pancreatitis caused by antimicrobials (eg, trimethoprim-sulfamethoxazole) or antiretroviral drugs (eg, didanosine) (Table 8.1). Infectious causes of hepatitis include viral,[2] bacterial, parasitic, and fungal pathogens (Table 8.2) that manifest as hepatitis, granulomatous hepatitis, cholangitis, or liver abscess (Fig. 8.1).

Acute Enteritis

Host responses leading to different clinical manifestations among the three major syndromes of acute enteric infections include: (1) Secretory diarrhea characterized by no fever or only low-grade fever, no white blood cells in stool sample and usually caused by *Vibrio cholerae*, Enterotoxigenic *Escherichia coli*, Enteroaggregative *E. coli* or by Enterohemoryhagic *E. coli*; (2) Inflammatory diarrhea caused by *Campylobacter jejuni*, *Shigella* app., nontyphoidal *Salmonella* serotypes (some may also cause bacteremia), and Enteroinvasive *E. coli*. During this type of enteritis, there is no associated fever but there is important presence of neutrophils in stool samples; and (3) Invasive disease in the form of bacteremia or enteric fever and caused by Typhoidal Salmonella serotypes, *Yersinia* spp., or *Brucella* spp.

Chronic Enteritis

Chronic infections of the small intestine cause significant morbidity and mortality globally. The most important clinical syndromes produced by chronic enteric infections consist of malabsorption with its associated complications,

Core Concepts in Clinical Infectious Diseases (CCCID). http://dx.doi.org/10.1016/B978-0-12-804423-0.00008-1

79

TABLE 8.1 Clinical Spectrum and Differential Diagnosis of Pancreatic Syndromes

Category	Etiology	Core concepts
Acute pancreatitis[a]	Biliary obstruction	Choledocholithiasis (up to 40% of cases)
	Chronic alcohol use	Up to 30–35% of cases
	Drug induced	Thiazide diuretics, furosemide, pentamidine, sulfonamides, tetracycline, valproic acid, azathioprine, didanosine, metronidazole, cimetidine, erythromycin
	Metabolic	Hypercalcemia, Hypertrygliceridemia
	Infectious	Viral (mumps, Coxsackievirus B4 (CB4-P and CB4-V, Hepatitis B Virus, cytomegalovirus, Herpes simplex virus, Varicella–Zoster virus, HIV)
		Bacterial (*Mycoplasma pneumoniae*, leptospirosis, tuberculosis, *S. Typhi*, *Yersinia enterocolitica*, *Yersinia pseudotuberculosis*, brucellosis, *Legionella pneumophila*, *Nocardia* spp., *Mycobacterium avium-intracellulare*)
		Fungal (*Candida* spp., *Cryptococcus neoformans*)
		Parasitic (*Ascaris lumbricoides* migration through the biliary tract, *Chlonorchis sinensis*, *Fasciola hepatica*, *Opistorchis* sp., and *Dicrocoelium dendritycum*, *Cryptosporidium*)
	HIV/AIDS associated	(*Candida*, *Cryptococcus neoformans*, *Mycobacterium avium-intracellulare*, tuberculosis, Cytomegalovirus, *Pneumocystis jiroveci*, *Leishmania donovani*, *Cryptosporidium*, drug-induced (didanosine, pentavalent antimonials), Kaposi's sarcoma, lymphoma)
	Toxins	Scorpion or snake bites
	Ischemia/vasculitis	
	Tumor related	
Chronic pancreatitis[b]	Toxic metabolic	Uremia, alcohol, hypercalcemia, hyperlipidemia
	Idiopathic	Tropical calcific pancreatitis and fibrocalculous pancreatic diabetes
	Genetic	Cationic trypsinogen (autosomal dominant) Mutations of the cystic fibrosis transmembrane conductance regulator (CFTR), serine peptidases inhibitor (SPINK1), cationic trypsinogen, alpha1-antitrypsin deficiency

TABLE 8.1 Clinical Spectrum and Differential Diagnosis of Pancreatic Syndromes (*cont.*)

Category	Etiology	Core concepts
	Autoimmune/ inflammatory	IgG4-related disease, inflammatory bowel disease, primary biliary cirrhosis
	Recurrent and severe acute pancreatitis	Post irradiation, postnecrotic (severe acute pancreatitis), ischemia
		IgG4-related disease
	Obstructive	Pancreas divisum, disorders of the sphincter, duct obstruction caused by neoplasias
Pancreatic masses	Neoplasms of the exocrine pancreas	Pancreatic ductal carcinoma (>75%)
		Acinar cell carcinomas
		Adenosquamous Carcinomas
		Colloid carcinomas
		Hepatoid carcinomas
		Pancreatic intraepithelial neoplasia
		Intraductal papillary Mucinous neoplasms (IPMNs)
		Mucinous cystic neoplasms
		Pancreatoblastomas
		Serous cystadenomas
		Signet ring cell carcinoma
		Solid-pseudopapillary Neoplasm
		Undifferentiated Carcinomas
		Undifferentiated carcinoma with osteoclast-like giant cells
	Neoplasms of the endocrine pancreas	Neuroendocrine tumors (insulinomas, glucagonomas)
	Infections/ inflammatory disease mimicking neoplasms	Autoimmune pancreatitis (IgG4-related disease) [c]
		Tuberculosis of the pancreas[d]
		Pancreatic pseudocyst[e,f]

[a]*Quinlan JD. Acute pancreatitis. Am Fam Physician 2014;90(9):632–639.*
[b]*Nair RJ, Miller MR. Chronic pancreatitis. Am Fam Physician 2007;76:1679–1688.*
[c]*Kanisawa T, Zen Y, Pillai S, Stone JH. IgG4-related disease. Lancet 2015;385(9976):1460–1471.*
[d]*Franco-Paredes C, Leonard M, Jurado R, Blumberg HM, Smith R. Tuberculosis of the pancreas mimicking carcinoma: report of two cases and review of the literature. Am J Med Sci 2002;323(1):54–58.*
[e]*Whitcomb DC. Acute pancreatitis. N Engl J Med 2006;354:2142–2150.*
[f]*Pseudocyts is a cyst or collection of fluid not contained within an enclosed membrane or sac of its own epithelium lining. A pancreatic pseudocyst develops inside pancreatic tissue and surrounded fibrous connective tissue and contains semisolid tissue and high levels of pancreatic enzymes.*

TABLE 8.2 Differential Diagnosis and Clinical Spectrum of Hepatitis

Category	Differential diagnosis	Core concepts
Viral hepatitis	Hepatitis E virus (HEV)[a]	The four genotypes of HEV (1–4) fall into two clinical syndromes: (1) Epidemic hepatitis associated with waterborne transmission with human viruses (genotypes 1–2) and (2) Autochtonous type due to genotypes 3–4 which are swine viruses domestic and wild pigs and accidentally infect humans
	Hepatitis B virus	Acute and chronic hepatitis B Hepatocarcinoma, cirrhosis
	Hepatitis C virus	Acute and chronic hepatitis C Complications: hepatocarcinoma, cirrhosis
	Hepatitis D virus	Superinfection or Coinfection with hepatitis B
	Hepatitis A virus	Sometimes fulminant hepatitis, sometimes may cause meningitis or relapse in 15% of cases
Other viruses	Epstein–Barr virus Cytomegalovirus	Infectious Mononucleosis and Post-Traumatic Lymphroliferative Disorder and may have a cholestasis pattern[b]
	Herpes simplex virus	Sometimes fulminant hepatitis in pregnant women and other immunosuppressive conditions
	Measles HIV	In some cases, patients may develop cirrhosis associated to the use of the antiretroviral drug DDI (didanosine)
Parasitic	Trematodes	*Schistosoma mansoni* reaches the liver via the portal vein where it induces *Fasciola hepatica* reaches the liver and biliary tract after reaching the abdominal cavity after penetrating the intestinal wall *Clonorchis sinensis* and *Opistorchis viverrini* cause biliary tract disease *Opistorchis viverrini* is associated with cholangiocarcinoma
Spirochetes	*Treponema pallidum*	Spirochetes reach the liver during the secondary stage of syphilis
	Leptospira interrogans	Biphasic febrile illness, cholestasis-hepatitis, and acute renal failure

TABLE 8.2 Differential Diagnosis and Clinical Spectrum of Hepatitis (*cont.*)

Category	Differential diagnosis	Core concepts
Fungal	*Candida albicans*[c]	Hepatosplenic candidiasis in patients postneutropenic fever
	Coccidiodes immitis	
	Cryptococcus neoformans	
	Histoplasma capsulatum	Sometimes associated with hemophagocytic syndrome
	Histoplasma dubosii	Sometimes associated with hemophagocytic syndrome
Bacterial	*Klebisella pneumoniae* invasive syndrome	Mucoid strain with metastatic infection to other sites (eg, endophtalmitis)
	Mycobacterium tuberculosis	Acute disseminated tuberculosis
		Miliary tuberculosis
		Obstructive jaundice due to porta hepatis lymphadenopathy or hepatic infiltration
	Listeria monocytogenes	Associated with bacteremia, foodborne and may cause liver abscess
	Mycobacterium avium-intracellulare	Granulomatous hepatitis
	Brucella mellitensis	Granulomatous hepatitis
	Actinomyces israelii	Hepatic infiltration
		Cytokine mediated cholestasis
	Sepsis	
Rickettsial	*Tickborne*	
	Ehrlichia chaffeensis Ehrlichia ewingii	Human granulocytic rhrlichiosis
	Rickettsia ricketsii	Rocky Mountain spotted fever
	Aerosolized from animal exposure	
	Coxiella burnetti	Q fever
Hemophagocytic syndrome	Infection-associated hemophagocytic syndrome	Hepatic infiltration
		Associated Infections:
		Epstein–Barr virus
		HIV
		Histoplasmosis
		Active tuberculosis
Granulomatous diseases	Sarcoidosis	Affected in >20% of patients with sarcoidosis. Most of these cases present with a cholestasis pattern

(*Continued*)

TABLE 8.2 Differential Diagnosis and Clinical Spectrum of Hepatitis (*cont.*)

Category	Differential diagnosis	Core concepts
Hepatic amyloidosis	AA amyloidosis (secondary)	Secondary to osteomyelitis or tuberculosis, may present with a cholestasis pattern due to hepatic infiltration
	AL amyloidosis (primary)	Multiple Myeloma or Waldenström macroglobulinemia
Neoplasias	Hodgkin's disease and Non-Hodgkin's lymphomas	Cytokine-mediated pattern of cholestasis plus hepatic infiltration
	Stauffer syndrome	Cytokine-mediated pattern of cholestasis
Autoimmune/ inflammatory diseases	IgG-4-related disease Sjögren's syndrome	Cholestasis pattern Obstructive jaundice or associated with primary sclerosing cholangitis or primary biliary cirrhosis
	Systemic sclerosis Henoch–Schönlein purpura	Obstructive jaundice and autoimmune small vessel vasculitis
	Primary biliary cirrhosis	Obstructive jaundice
	Crohn's disease	Granulomatous hepatitis
Congestive hepatopathy	Right sided heart failure Constrictive pericarditis	May lead to ascites, splenomegaly, and encephalopathy. Concomitant ischemic hepatitis may lead to severe liver injury
HIV associated[c]	Noncirrhotic portal hypertension	Some cases associated with didanosine
	Viral	Viral hepatitis (B and C), EBV, CMV, HSV-1/2, HHV-6
	Drug induced	Isoniazid and rifampin Pyrazinamide Darunavir Ritonavir Didanosine
	Parasitic	Schistosomiasis Visceral leishmaniasis
	Nonalcoholic steatohepatitis	
	HIV colangiopathy	Some cases of colangiopathy caused by Cytomegalovirus or *Cryptosporidium*

[a]*Epidemic HEV has a high attack rate among adolescents and young adults with high mortality in pregnant women. There is an HEV vaccine approved in China. Autochtonous (genotypes 3 and 4) cause high mortality among adult men with high neurologic sequelae and it may cause chronic hepatitis E.*
[b]*DeLemos AS, Friedman LS. Systemic causes of cholestasis. Clin Liver Dis 2013;17(2):301–317.*
[c]*Mendizabal M, Craviotto S, Chen T, Silva MO, Reddy KR. Noncirrhotic portal hypertension: another cause of liver disease in HIV patients. Ann Hepatol 2009;8(4):390–395; Cainelli F. Human immunodeficiency virus infection and the liver. World J Hepatol 2012;4(3):91–98.*

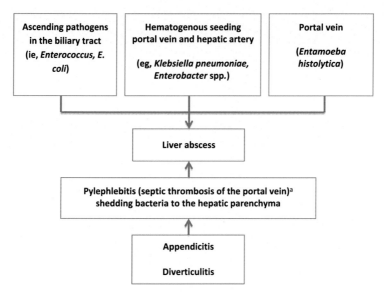

FIGURE 8.1 Mechanisms in the pathogenesis of liver abscess. (*ªMorris MA, Regenbogen SE, Hardiman KM, Hendren S. Sigmoid diverticulitis. A systematic review. JAMA 2014;311(3):287–297; Choudhry AJ, Baghdadi YMK, Amr MA, Alzghari MJ, Jenkins DH, Zielinski MD. Pylephebitis: a review of 95 cases. J Gastrointest Surg 2015; doi: 10.1007/s11605-015-2875-3)*

gastrointestinal hemorrhage, perforation peritonitis, and other systemic complications. The most important causes of chronic enteric infections include: (1) giardiasis or other enteric pathogens triggering or unmasking subclinical celiac disease; (2) tropical sprue; (3) tropical enteropathy; (4) Whipple's disease by the causative organism *Tropheryma whippleii*; (5) intestinal tuberculosis which sometimes, similarly to typhoid fever, may lead to gastrointestinal hemorrhage or perforation peritonitis; (6) fungal infections such as histoplasmosis, aspergillosis, candidiasis, and others.

Typhoid fever and paratyphoid fever (enteric fever) remain as important pathogens in many settings. In addition, nontyphoidal salmonellosis is an important source of morbidity and mortality among patients with HIV/AIDS or malnourished (Fig. 8.2).

Many insults targeting the liver may produce a fulminant course characterized by coagulopathy and encephalopathy (Table 8.3). Alternatively, a chronic hepatic fibrosis is a common response to the long-term injury to the liver. The hepatic lipocyte or Ito cell is located in the perisinusoidal space if it along with Disse is responsible for most of the extracellular matrix production and deposition. Cirrhosis of the liver is associated with portal hypertension and ascites. Spontaneous bacterial peritonitis is an important source of sepsis in patients with portal hypertension and ascites. Inflammatory or infectious causes of aortitis are important to consider in the differential diagnosis of abdominal pain in patients with underlying systemic illness including vasculitis or autoimmune or inflammatory diseases.[3]

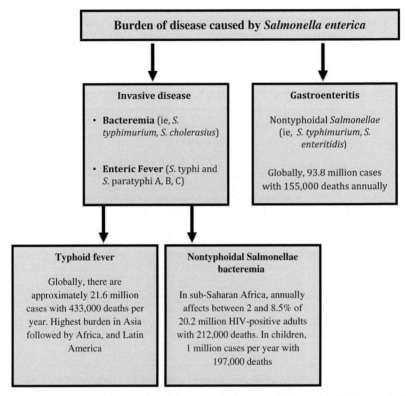

FIGURE 8.2   Enteric Fever (Typhoid Fever and Paratyphoid Fever) and Non-Typhoidal Salmonellosis.

TABLE 8.3 Differential Diagnosis of Acute Liver Failure[a,b]

Category	Etiology
Toxins	Carbon tetrachloride *Amanita phalloides* Phosphorus
Viral hepatitis	Herpes simplex Hepatitis A Hepatitis B/Hepatitis D superinfection
	Hepatitis B Hepatitis C Herpes simplex virus Dengue virus Epstein–Barr virus Yellow fever Parvovirus B19 Human herpes virus-6 (HHV-6) Cytomegalovirus Parainfluenza

TABLE 8.3 Differential Diagnosis of Acute Liver Failure[a,b] (*cont.*)

Category	Etiology
Vascular	Ischemia Venoocclusive disease Heat stroke Budd–Chiari syndrome
Metabolic	Wilson's disease Reye's syndrome Acute fatty liver of pregnancy Nonalcoholic steatohepatitis Tyrosinemia Galactosemia Sepsis
Drug related	Dose dependent Acetaminophen, isoniazid, tetracycline, *Amanita Phalloides* Synergistic Ethanol plus acetaminophen Barbiturate plus acetaminophen Isoniazid plus rifampicin Drug reaction eosinophilic systemic syndrome
Autoimmune	Autoimmune hepatitis Primary biliary cirrhosis Primary sclerosing cholangitis associated with inflammatory bowel disease

[a]*Acute liver failure is defined by a hepatic injury associated with encephalopathy and coagulopathy.*
[b]*In the case of spontaneous bacterial peritonitis associated with ascites in patients with cirrhosis causing portal hypertension, abdominal paracentesis is crucial in their evaluation. Spontaneous bacterial peritonitis (SBP) should be considered in a patient with ascites presenting with sepsis or acute clinical worsening without a clear clinical explanation. Ascitic fluid should be obtained to perform gram staining and culture (it is recommended to use blood culture bottles to improve sensitivity) with cell counts (more than 500 white blood cells or more than 250 Polymorphonuclears (PMNs) are considered as highly suggestive of SBP.*
Lee WM. Acute liver failure. N Engl J Med 1993;**329**(25):1862–1871.

REFERENCES

1. Working Group IAP/APA Acute Pancreatitis Guidelines. IAP/APA evidence-based guidelines for the management of acute pancreatitis. *Pancreatology* 2013;**13**:e1–e15.
2. Lok ASF, McMahon BJ. Chronic hepatitis B. *Hepatology* 2007;**45**:507–39.
3. Nay J, Menias CO, Mellnick VM, Balfe DM. Gastrointestinal manifestations of systemic disease: a multimodality review. *Abdom Imaging* 2015;**40**:1926–43.

Chapter 9

Genitourinary Infections

DIAGNOSTIC APPROACH TO GENITOURINARY INFECTIONS AND INFLAMMATORY INFECTIONS

Urinary Tract Syndromes

Urinary tract infections (UTI) may involve the lower or upper tracts, or both, and can therefore involve the urethra, bladder, ureters, kidneys, and perinephric space.[1–3] This group of infections manifest through a clinical spectrum of clinical syndromes that ranges from asymptomatic bacteriuria, to sterile pyuria, to symptomatic UTI (complicated and uncomplicated), and to sepsis associated with UTI.[4] Complicated UTI refers to having a symptomatic UTI in patients with any of the following criteria: (1) presence of a functional or structural abnormality; (2) undergone recent urinary-tract instrumentation; (3) presence of a significant systemic condition associated with immunosuppression such as organ transplantation, uncontrolled diabetes mellitus, malignancy undergoing chemotherapy, or renal insufficiency.[2]

The clinical spectrum and differential diagnosis of uncomplicated and complicated UTI is depicted in Table 9.1[3]. Conditions associated with sterile pyuria are noted in Table 9.2. Infections in the kidney and perinephric space include a variety of presentations of intrarenal abscesses and perirenal abscesses[2] (Table 9.3).

Sexually Transmitted Diseases and Syndromes

The group of sexually transmitted diseases includes a diverse group of organisms including bacterial, viral, fungal, and parasitic pathogens capable of causing distinct clinical syndromes and infections including[4]: (1) genital, anal, or perianal ulcers (Table 9.4); (2) diseases characterized by urethritis and cervicitis (Table 9.5), (3) vaginal discharge (Table 9.6); (4) pelvic inflammatory disease (Table 9.7); (5) epididimytis, proctitis, anogenital warts, and anal carcinomas (Table 9.8). Syphilis has been called "the great imitator" due to its ability to cause a myriad of clinical presentations and a summary of the urogenital and systemic entities are noted in Table 9.9. Other considerations within the spectrum of sexually transmitted diseases include some cases of HIV, HTLV-1, hepatitis B virus infection, hepatitis C virus infection, and hepatitis A virus infection. Some ectoparasitosis such as lice and scabies may also be sexually acquired.[5]

Core Concepts in Clinical Infectious Diseases (CCCID). http://dx.doi.org/10.1016/B978-0-12-804423-0.00009-3

TABLE 9.1 Clinical Approach to Uncomplicated and Complicated Urinary Tract Infections[a]

Uncomplicated urinary tract infections	Complicated urinary tract infections
This category comprises episodes of acute cystitis and pyelonephritis taking place in healthy nonpregnant women, premenopausal with no history suggest of an abnormal urinary tract	Anyone with anatomical, functional, or metabolic abnormalities that may increase the risk of poor clinical outcomes including nephrolithiasis, renal insufficiency, diabetes mellitus, neurogenic bladder, bladder outlet obstruction syndrome, pregnancy, or severe immunosuppression, as well as recent urinary tract instrumentation (cystoscopy, stent placement, endoscopic procedures, biopsy of the prostate, etc.) or that present with sepsis
Most common implicated pathogens include *Escherichia coli, Klebisella pneumoniae, Staphylococcus saprophyticus, Enterococcus faecalis,* group B streptococci	
Acute uncomplicated cystitis rarely progresses to severe disease, even if untreated and thus the goal is to ameliorate symptoms	
First line outpatient antimicrobial treatment include nitrofurantoin, trimethoprim-sulfamethoxazole, fosfomycin, or pivmecillinam[b]	Urianalysis and urine culture are indicated
Recurrent cystitis requires prophylactic antimicrobial therapy when nonantimicrobial preventive strategies are not effective	Symptomatic UTI in older women including community-dwelling and nursing home residents with our without urinary-indwelling catheters have a high rate of chronic genitourinary symptoms and therefore when ruling urinary tract infections, laboratory testing should include urianalysis and urine culture[c]
Fluoroquinolones are first-line agent for empirical treatment of pyelonephritis but second-line agent for the empiric treatment of cystitis	These urinary studies should only be performed if patient's symptoms worsen acutely (ie, acute change in mental status) and not explained by other reasons
Recurrent cystitis is often treated successfully with every 10-day 3-g therapy with fosfomycin	The presence of foul smelling urine, or change in the turbidity of the urine are clinically helpful in this particular age group, particularly with long-term urinary catheter use where diagnosing UTI, is often a major challenge
	Hospitalized individuals with complicate UTI should receive broad-spectrum coverage and then narrow treatment according to culture results

UTI, Urinary tract infections.
[a]*Distinguishing between uncomplicated and complicated UTI is used to guide the choice and duration of antimicrobial therapy, with broader-spectrum antimicrobials and longer courses of treatment for individuals suffering from a complicated UTI. This classification is helpful but one that stratifies patients into multiple homogeneous categories may provide better clinical information for empiric and specific management (Hooton TM. Uncomplicated urinary tract infection. N Engl J Med 2012;**366**(11):1028–1037).*
[b]*Antimicrobial resistance does not necessarily indicate a complicated UTI.*
[c]Mody L, Juthani-Mehta M. Urinary tract infections in older women. A clinical review. JAMA 2014;**311**(8):844–854.

TABLE 9.2 Differential Diagnosis of Sterile Pyuria[a,b]

Category	Etiology	Core concepts
Sexually transmitted diseases	*Chlamydia trachomatis* *Neisseria gonorrhoeae* *Mycoplasma genitalum* *Ureaplasma urealyticum* Herpes simplex virus (1 and 2)	Chlamydia infection is the most common cause of sterile pyuria
	Varicella–Zoster virus (VZV) Human papillomavirus (HPV)	VZV causes sterile pyuria in patients with cystitis when there is herpes zoster lumbosacral involvement with voiding dysfunction
	HIV/AIDS	Patients with advanced HIV/AIDS often have evidence of pyuria
Antibiotic use	Current use of antibiotics for UTI Recently treated urinary tract infection within the past 2 weeks	Leukocyturia may persist some time even after effective sterilization of the urinary tract with adequate antimicrobial therapy
Tuberculosis	Genitourinary tuberculosis	The genitourinary tract is the most common extrapulmonary site of tuberculosis after lymphatic; and may occur with concomitant active pulmonary tuberculosis in 4–8% of cases
Fungal infection	*Aspergillus* spp. *Cryptococcus neoformans,* *Blastomyces,* *Coccidiodes,* *Histoplasma* *Candida* spp. (*C. albicans, C. krusei, C. glabrata*)	Most common source is hematogenous but ascending infection is also possible
Gastrointestinal	Acute appendicitis	IF the appendix lies close to a ureter or the bladder and irritates these structures
Viral infections	BK polyoma virus CMV	Among individuals with kidney transplantation

(Continued)

TABLE 9.2 Differential Diagnosis of Sterile Pyuria[a,b] (cont.)

Category	Etiology	Core concepts
Parasitic	Schistosomiasis (*Schistosoma haematobium*)	In endemic areas schistosomiasis is a common cause of genitourinary disease, particularly among women
	Trichomoniasis (*Trichomonas vaginalis*)	A highly prevalent infection in some parts of the United States
Urinary catheters	Presence or recent use of a urinary catheter	
Urinary tract instrumentation	Recent cystoscopy or urologic endoscopic procedures	Also, those with surgical mesh in the urethra or a retained stent
Pelvic radiation	Pelvic or genitourinary malignancies	
Nephrotic syndrome	Renal-vein thrombosis	Hypercoagulability due to loss of anticoagulant proteins
Interstitial nephritis and papillary necrosis	Drug-induced nephropathy (analgesic nephropathy)	Papillary necrosis tends to occur in patients with diabetes mellitus
Drug-induced mucosal involvement	Stevens–Johnson's/toxic epidermic necrolysis Erythema multiforme	
Inflammatory	Kawasaki's disease Interstitial cystitis Reiter's syndrome (reactive arthritis)	

[a]*Pyuria is defined as the presence of 10 or more white cells per cubic millimeter in a urine specimen, three or more white cells per high-power field of unspun urine, or a positive result on Gram-staining of an unspun urine specimen, or a urinary dipstick test that is positive for leukocyte esterase (Wise GJ, Schlegel PN. Sterile pyuria. N Engl J Med 2015;**372**(11):1048–1054).*
[b]*Sterile pyuria is the persistent finding of white cells in the urine in the absence of bacteria as determined through aerobic microbiologic techniques (urine cultured in blood agar and MacConkey agar plates) (Wise GJ, Schlegel PN. Sterile pyuria. N Engl J Med 2015;372(11):1048–1054).*

TABLE 9.3 Renal and Perirenal Infections and Inflammatory Syndromes[a]

Category	Diseases	Core concepts
Perinephric space	*Perirenal abscess*	Occurs in the perinephric fascia external to the capsule of the kidney between the renal capsule and Gerota's fascia
	Gram-negative perinephric abscess develops from a ruptured renal corticomedullary abscess	Usually as a result of extension of an intrarenal abscess into this area
	Staphylococcal perinephric abscess develops from a ruptured cortical abscess	Complication of a urinary tract infection or sometimes initiating events include hematogenous or regional lymphatic seeding from skin sites
	Associated conditions Diabetes mellitus	
	Caused by Gram-negative bacilli including *Klebsiella* spp., *E. coli, Enterobacter, Pseudomonas,* and *Proteus; Staphylococcus aureus, Streptococcus pneumoniae;* anaerobes such as *Bacteroides* spp., *Clostridium, and Actinomyces; Candida* or *M. tuberculosis*	Other inflammatory processes that may be the primary focus of spread of infection include appendicitis, diverticulitis, or perforated colon It can spread to cause a subphrenic abscess, an empyema, or a nephrobronchial fistula
Renal cortical	*Cortical abscess (renal carbuncle)*	Results from a primary focus of infection elsewhere in the body (osteomyelitis, bacteremia, cellulitis, or pyodermas leading to hematogenous spread to kidney
	Associated conditions Hemodialysis, intravenous drug use (IVDU), diabetes mellitus	Focus of infection is not found in one third of cases because manifestations from kidney involvement may take a few weeks
	Differential diagnosis includes renal carcinomas and treatment requires intravenous antibiotics and sometimes surgical evacuation depending on size and clinical course	Cortical microabscesses coalesce and enlarge forming a fluid-filled mass with a thick wall (most renal carbuncles are single lesions)

(Continued)

TABLE 9.3 Renal and Perirenal Infections and Inflammatory Syndromes[a] (*cont.*)

Category	Diseases	Core concepts
	Caused by *Staphylococcus aureus* in 90% of cases	Cortical abscesses may rupture into the renal capsule and form a perinephric abscess
Corticomedullar	*Corticomedullar abscess* Complication of bacteriuria and ascending infection associated with an underlying urinary tract abnormality including vesicoureteral reflux or urinary tract obstruction (tubular scarring from previous infections and renal calculi), genitourinary abnormalities associated with primary hyperparathyroidism, diabetes mellitus	Contains a spectrum of acute and chronic inflammatory processes: *Acute focal bacterial nephritis* (acute lobar nephronia or focal pyelonephritis): no abscess and it is an acute bacterial interstitial nephritis affecting a single renal lobe *Acute multifocal bacterial nephritis:* abscess formation and inflammatory infiltrate throughout the kidney
	Caused by Gram-negative bacilli including *Klebsiella* spp., *E. coli,* and *Proteus* sp.	*Emphysematous pyelonephritis:* it is a severe necrotizing acute multifocal bacterial nephritis with extraluminal and retroperitoneal gas (diabetes mellitus associated) Xantogranulomatous pyelonephritis: severe infection of the renal parenchyma with destruction of the renal parenchyma and replaced by granulomatous tissue containing lipid-laden foamy macrophages (most often caused by renal calculi)[b]
Parenchyma	Infected renal cyst Caused by Gram-negative bacilli infecting the cyst by ascending route	Spontaneous infection of preexisting solitary renal cysts but more often occurring in patients with polycystic kidney disease with a single or multiple cysts infected

TABLE 9.3 Renal and Perirenal Infections and Inflammatory Syndromes[a] **(cont.)**

Category	Diseases	Core concepts
Tuberculosis	Renal involvement can be indolent for more than 20 years and consisting of granuloma formation coalescing and developing into mass-like lesions with central necrosis and often rupturing into the draining calyx spreading infection into the renal pelvis and further distally	In renal tuberculosis, as the disease progresses, there is a fibrotic reaction causing stenosis and stricture formation of the calyceal infundibula leading to uneven caliectasis followed by calcium deposition Longstanding renal tuberculosis may result in renal parenchymal atrophy, hydronephrosis, and autonephrectomy Most common site of genitourinary involvement is the epididymis in men and fallopian tube involvement in women
Fungal infections of the kidney	Renal aspergillosis (*Aspergillus* spp.) *Candida* spp. (most commonly *C. albicans, C. glabrata)*	Manifesting as a complex cystic lesion/abscess among severely immunocompromised hosts Patients become infected via hematogenous route or ascending infection from the lower urinary tract *C. albicans* acquired from hematogenous route may cause multiple renal abscesses (as part of invasive candidiasis—see chapter: Bloodstream Infections). It may also be associated with fungus balls or mycetomas which are collections of inflammatory cells, fungus, necrotic or mucoid debris, and calculous matrix
Parasitic infections of the kidney	Renal echinoccosis (renal hydatid disease is usually unilateral)	Caused by the tapeworm *Echinococcus granulosus* with the liver and lung being the most commonly affected organs. Presents as large multiseptated cysts mimicking renal carcinoma If the cyst ruptures it may cause a severe system allergic reaction

[a]*Drainage of the abscesses and sometimes partial or complete nephrectomy, in addition to antibiotic therapy, are required for resolution.*
[b]*Renal malakoplakia is a chronic inflammatory process associated with E. coli that involves the urinary tract collecting system, most commonly the bladder. It occurs due to an abnormal macrophage function that prevents complete destruction of phagocytosed bacteria with the presence of intracellular inclusion bodies called Michaelis-Gutmann bodies.*

TABLE 9.4 Differential Diagnosis of Infectious and Non-Infectious Causes of Genital, Perianal or Anal Ulcers[a]

Category	Etiologies	Core concepts
Sexually transmitted diseases (STDs)	*Most frequent causes*	*Clinical description*
	Syphilis (*Treponema pallidum*)	Usually single, nontender, indurated edge, clean base, and nontender inguinal adenopathy (RPR and darkfield examination)
	Herpes simplex type 2 or type 1	Usually multiple, superficial, marked tenderness, soft edge, clean base, tender adenopathy (Tzanck smear, viral culture)
	Chancroid (*Haemophilus ducreyi*)	Starts as a tender erythematous papule followed by a pustule that ruputer and progresses to a painful ragged ulcer(s). Usually multiple ulcers, marked tenderness, soft edge, dirty base, tender and fluctuant adenopathy. The combination of a painful genital ulcer and tender suppurative inguinal adenopathy is highly suggestive of chancroid
	Less frequent causes	*Clinical description*
	Lymphogranuloma venereum (*Chlamydia trachomatis* serovars L_1, L_2, or L_3)	Usually single non-tender ulcer, soft edge, base is an eroded papule and prominent and tender inguinal adenopathy (positive serology complement fixation (titers $\geq$ 1:64 or microimmunofluorescence $\geq$1:256)
	Donovanosis (*Klebisella granulomatis*)	Also called granuloma inguinale, the disease is commonly characterized as painless, slowly progressive ulcerative lesions on the genitals or perineum without regional lymphadenopathy but pseudobuboes consisting of subcutaneous granulomas can be present. Lesions are vascular and can bleed (beefy red appearance). There may be extragenital infection involving the pelvis, bones, or the mouth (diagnosis requires visualization of dark-staining Donovan bodies on tissue crush preparation or biopsy

TABLE 9.4 Differential Diagnosis of Infectious and Non-Infectious Causes of Genital, Perianal or Anal Ulcers[a] (*cont.*)

Category	Etiologies	Core concepts
	HIV	Can be seen during early HIV-infection (acute retroviral syndrome)
	Protozoal	
	Entamoeba histolytica	Associated to rectal sexual activity
	Schistosoma haematobium	In highly endemic areas, it may be a co-factor in the acquisition or transmission of HIV[b]
Inflammatory	Behcet's disease	Behcet's disease requires meeting diagnostic criteria of recurrent oral aphtae and at least two other including genital apthae, arthritis, uveitis, cutaneous vasculitis, or meningitis
	Crohn's disease	Most cases have gastrointestinal involvement. However isolated cases of genital Crohn's disease have been reported
	Psoriasis	Disease present in other sites and extending into genital area
Neoplastic	Erythroplasia of Queyrat (Bowen disease of the glans penis)	In situ squamous cell carcinoma of the penis almost exclusively in uncircumcised men; it can also describe squamous cell carcinoma in situ of the labia minora, vestibule, vulva, or labia majora
	Squamous cell carcinoma	
Drug reaction	Recurrent erythema multiforme (drug-induced or infectious-triggered)	Usually present with oral mucosa affection and occurs sometimes after an episode of herpes simplex 1 or 2 reactivation
	Acute vulva fixed drug eruption	Most frequently associated with anti-inflammatory drugs and sulfa drugs, tetracyclines, barbiturates
Nonsexually acquired genital ulcer[c]	Occurring after pharyngitis, upper viral infection or gastroenteritis	May respond to oral doxycycline and topical steroids

(Continued)

TABLE 9.4 Differential Diagnosis of Infectious and Non-Infectious Causes of Genital, Perianal or Anal Ulcers[a] (cont.)

Category	Etiologies	Core concepts
Postinfectious (reactive) aphtous ulcers (previously named complex aphtous ulcer)	Epstein–Barr virus infection (Lipshütz ulcer) usually presenting in young women	
Trauma	Factitial	Present in uncommon sites and sometimes associated with psychiatric illness (eg, schizophrenia)
	Trauma during sexual intercourse	

[a]*Genital, anal, or perianal lesions and chancroid have been associated with HIV acquisition and transmission. The diagnostic workup of genital, anal, or perianal ulcers should include: darkfield examination, syphilis serology, or PCR testing if available; culture or PCR for HSV and serologic testing for type-specific HSV antibody; specific culture for Haemophilus ducreyi or PCR testing if available. It is important to consider LGV serological testing. Some individuals may have more than one kind of infectious cause of genital ulcers.*
[b]*Genital manifestations of schistosoma mansoni in women: important but neglected. Mem Inst Oswaldo Cruz 1998;**93**(Suppl 1):127–133.*
[c]*Dixit S, Bradford J, Fischer G. Management of nonsexually acquired genital ulceration using oral and topical corticosteroids followed by doxycycline prophylaxis. J Am Acad Dermatol 2013;**68**:797–802.*

TABLE 9.5 Differential Diagnosis of Urethritis and Cervicitis[a]

Category[b]	Diseases	Key clinical considerations
Urethritis	Infectious	
	Bacterial	*Neisseria gonorrhaoeae* *Chlamydia trachomatis* *Mycoplasma genitalum* (may also cause prostatitis) Enteric bacteria (associated with insertive anal intercourse)
	Parasitic viral	*Trichomonas vaginalis* Herpes simplex Epstein–Barr virus
	Noninfectious	Trauma Reiter's syndrome (part of reactive arthritis syndrome conjunctivitis, sterile urethritis, and arthritis) Allergic irritation (latex in condoms) Use of genital antiseptics can cause irritation Drug reactions: erythema multiforme or during Stevens–Johnson's syndrome with mucosal involvement
Cervicitis[c]	Cervicitis frequently is asymptomatic	Most common etiologies include *Neisseria gonorrhoeae, Chlamydia trachomatis, T. vaginalis,* and Herpes Simplex Virus
	Some women complain of an abnormal vaginal discharge and intermenstrual vaginal bleeding sometimes occurring after sexual intercourse[d]	Women with cervicitis should be tested for bacterial vaginosis and should be assessed for the clinical presence of pelvic inflammatory disease

[a]*Centers for Disease Control and Prevention. Sexually transmitted diseases treatment guidelines, 2015. MMWR 2015;**64**(3):1–135.*
[b]*Urethritis is caused by urethral inflammation and manifest with dysuria, urethral pruritus; and mucoid, mucopurulent, or purulent discharge.*
[c]*Cervicitis is characterized by purulent of mucopurulent endocervical exudate visible in the endocervical canal or on an swab specimen and/or sustained endocervical bleeding easily induced by gentle passage of a cotton swab through the cervix os (Centers for Disease Control and Prevention. Sexually transmitted diseases treatment guidelines, 2015. MMWR 2015;**64**(3):1–135).*
[d]*Leukorrhea (≥10 white cells per high-power field on microscopic examination of vaginal fluid has been associated with chlamydial and gonococcal infection of the cervix.*

TABLE 9.6 Differential Diagnosis of Vaginal Discharge

Diseases	Core concepts
Bacterial vaginosis	Characterized by the replacement of vaginal bacterial flora (*Lactobacillus* sp. that produces hydrogen peroxide) by an overgrowth of anaerobic bacteria including *Prevotella* spp., *Mobiluncus* sp., *G. vaginalis*, *Ureaplasma*, *Mycoplasma*, and other anaerobes The pH of vaginal secretions is elevated $\geq$4.5 with bacterial vaginosis or trichomosiasis; application of 10% KOH solution to a vaginal discharge specimen may emit an amine odor suggests either bacterial vaginosis or trichomoniasis; saline solution specimen may demonstate trichomonads or clue cells (associated with bacterial vaginosis) It is associated with having multiple male or female partners, a new sex partner, douching, lack of condom use, and lack of vaginal lactobacilli Women with this condition are at increased risk for the acquisition of HIV, gonorrhoea, chlamydia, and herpes simplex virus-2
Candidiasis	Vulvovaginal candidiasis is caused mainly by *C. albicans*, followed by *C. glabrata* In addition to abnormal vaginal discharge, uncomplicated vulvovaginitis clinical presentation includes pruritus, vaginal soreness, dyspareunia, dysuria and usually responds to a short-course topical formulation of antifungal formulation or single dose of oral fluconazole Complicated disease is manifested as recurrent disease or severe manifestations including extensive vulvar erythema, edema, excoriation and fissure formation
Trichomoniasis	Most prevalent nonviral sexually transmitted infection in the United States and most cases occur among African American women and may cause diffuse, malodorous, yellow–green vaginal discharge with or without vulvar irritation Men may have urethritis, epididymitis, or prostatitis due to trichomoniasis
Cervicitis	As described in Table 9.5, cervicitis may be associated with vaginal discharge

TABLE 9.7 Clinical Spectrum of Pelvic Inflammatory Syndromes[a]

Category	Etiology	Core concepts
Acute pelvic inflammatory disease (PID) comprises a spectrum of inflammatory disorders of the upper female genital tract[b]: • Endometritis • Salpingitis • Tuboovarian abscess • Pelvic peritonitis	Associated with bacterial vaginosis Associated with cervical pathogens Other pathogens *Staphylococcus aureus, Haemophilus influenza, Streptococcus pneumoniae, Streptococcus pyogenes, Streptococcus agalactiae, Escherichia coli, Bacteroides fragilis*	Symptoms occurring for less than 30 with inflammation spreading from the vagina or cervix to the upper genital tract Pelvic tenderness and inflammation of the lower genital tract an manifesting as cervical motion tenderness, uterine tenderness, or adnexal tenderness
Chronic	*Mycobacterium tuberculosis* and *Actinomyces* spp.	Patients become infected via hematogenous dissemination or contiguous renal tuberculosis Patients most commonly present with infertility secondary to fallopian tube involvement and tuboovarian abscess may also develop. The endometrium is involved in more than 50% of patients with fallopian tube involvement
Fitz–Hugh curtis	*Neisseria gonorrhoeae Chlamydia trachomatis*	Right-upper quadrant pain caused by inflammation in the liver capsule with adhesions occurring in some individuals with acute pelvic inflammation
Subacute	*Neisseria gonorrhoeae Chlamydia trachomatis*	Clinically silent spread of infection from the lower genital tract
Acute PID concomitantly with disseminated gonococcal infection	*Neisseria gonorrhoeae*	Arthritis, cutaneous lesions and pelvic inflammatory symptoms

[a]*Preventing, diagnosis, and appropriately treating pelvic inflammatory disease is crucial given its frequent complications including ectopic pregnancy, tuboovarian abscess, infertility, and chronic pelvic pain (Brunhan RC, Gottlieb SL, Paavonen J. Pelvic inflammatory disease. N Engl J Med 2015;**372**(21):2039–2048).*

TABLE 9.8 Clinical Spectrum of Disease and Differential Diagnosis of Epididymitis, Proctitis, and Anogenital Warts/Carcinomas[a]

Category	Etiology	Core concepts
Epididymitis[b]	Acute epididymitis	
	Sexually active men of the age less than 35 years have C. trachomatis or N. gonorrhoeae or due to E. coli due to insertive anal intercourse	Frequently associated with urethritis which may be symptomatic or not; most frequently unilateral
	Men of more than 35 years of age with no history or anal insertive intercourse, the most common mechanism is bladder outlet obstruction (ie, benign prostatic hyperplasia) and bacteriuria seeding the epididymus and Gram-negative bacilli are frequently identified	In older men, epididymitis may also be caused by prostate biopsy, recent instrumentation of the urinary tract, systemic diseases including diabetes mellitus or immunosuppression
		Fournier's gangrene is often associated with epididymitis
	Chronic epididymitis	
	More than 6 week history of symptoms and signs (swelling and pain)	Most commonly caused by granulomatous diseases such as tuberculosis or brucellosis
		Some patients may develop chronic noninfectious epididymitis which may have an autoimmune or reactive etiology
Anogenital warts	There are more than 100 types of human papillomavirus (>40 can affect the genital area)	Oncogenic high-risk HPV infection such as HPV-16 and 18 causes most cervical, penile, vulvar, vaginal, anal and oropharyngeal cancers and precancerous lesions
	Persistent infection with oncogenic types of HPV has a causal role in nearly every cervical carcinomas, and in many vulvar, vaginal, penile, anal, and oropharyngeal carcinomas	Oncogenic low-risk HPV infection (HPV 6 and 11) causes recurrent respiratory papillomatosis and genital warts

TABLE 9.8 Clinical Spectrum of Disease and Differential Diagnosis of Epididymitis, Proctitis, and Anogenital Warts/Carcinomas[a] (*cont.*)

Category	Etiology	Core concepts
	HPV types 16, 18, 31, 33, and 35 are also occasionally found in anogenital warts and can be associated with high-grade squamous intraepithelial lesions (HSIL)	Only recommended routine screening for HPV-associated cancers is for cervical carcinoma. This is crucial in patients with HIV-infection[c]
Sexually transmitted gastrointestinal syndromes	Proctitis	Inflammation of the rectum associated with anorectal pain, tenesmus, or rectal discharge (caused by *N. gonorrhoeae, C. trachomatis* (including lymphogranuloma venereum serovars L1, L2, L3), *T. pallidum*, and HSV-2. Herpes proctitis may present with severe symptoms)
	Proctocolitis	Proctocolitis is associated with symptoms of proctitis and diarrhea, abdominal cramps, and inflammation of the colonic mucosa extending to 12 cm above the anus (caused by *Campylobacter* spp, *Shigella* spp, *Entamoeba histolytica* spp, and lymphogranuloma serovars of *C. trachomatis*). Among immunocompromised hosts, CMV or other opportunistic pathogens may be involved
	Enteritis	Diarrhea and abdominal cramping without signs of proctitis or proctocolitis. *Giardia lamblia* is most frequently implicated but other pathogens include CMV, *Mycobacerium avium-intarcellulare*, *Salmonella* spp., *Shigella* spp., *Campylobacter* sp., *Cryptosporidium, Microsporidium*, or Isospora

(Continued)

TABLE 9.8 Clinical Spectrum of Disease and Differential Diagnosis of Epididymitis, Proctitis, and Anogenital Warts/Carcinomas[a] (cont.)

Category	Etiology	Core concepts
		Outbreaks of *Shigella flexneri* serotype 3a and *Shigella sonnei* have been reported in men who have sex with men

[a]*Centers for Disease Control and Prevention. Sexually transmitted diseases treatment guidelines, 2015. MMWR 2015;**64**(3):1–135.*
[b]*Acute epididymitis is a clinical syndrome that comprises inflammation of the epididymus that lasts less than 6 weeks and characterized by swelling and pain of the testicular area. Sometimes the testicles are involved and thus the term epididymoorchitis. Testicular torsion must be always ruled out in men with sudden onset of scrotal swelling and pain.*
[c]*HPV vaccines are administered as a three-dose series of intramuscular injections over a 6-month period. For girls, either bivalent or quadrivalent vaccines should be offered routinely at ages 11–12 years and can be administered beginning at age 9; girls and women aged 13–26 years who have not started or completed the vaccine series should receive the vaccine. The quadrivalent or 9-valent HPV vaccine is recommended for boys aged 11–12 years but they can start vaccination at age 9; and those 13–21 who have not completed the schedule or have not received the vaccine, should receive the vaccine. For previously unvaccinated, immunocompromised hosts including HIV, and men-who have sex with men, vaccination is recommended up to age 26 (Centers for Disease Control and Prevention. Sexually transmitted diseases treatment guidelines, 2015. MMWR 2015;**64**(3):1–135).*

TABLE 9.9 Clinical Spectrum of Syphilis[a]

Diseases	Core concepts
Primary syphilis	Chancre (clean base ulcer indurated and usually single) associated with painless regional adenopathy usually presents in 3 weeks (range 3–90 days) Ulcer may be in the oral cavity, perianal, anal, or genital areas May be associated with neurosyphilis or may also, albeit rarely, with secondary syphilis
Secondary syphilis	Occurring 2–12 weeks from exposure (2 weeks–6 months) and represents systemic dissemination of *Treponema pallidum* Characteristic rash is usually papulo-squamous rash diffuse that can involve palms, soles, scalp, mucocutaneous lesions, fever, malaise, lymphadenopathy, mucosal lesions, condyloma lata,[b] alopecia, meningitis, headaches, tinnitus
Malignant syphilis (lues maligna)	Represents a severe form of secondary syphilis causing an nodular-ulcerative variant The rash manifests as pustules, nodules, or ulcers with or without mucosal involvement

TABLE 9.9 Clinical Spectrum of Syphilis[a] (cont.)

Diseases	Core concepts
	Histopathology shows a dearth of spirochetes with Warthin–Starry stains associated with a lymphocytic infiltration with predominance of plasma cells in the upper and middle dermis, superficial and deep vessels reveal a significant perivascular infiltrate, endothelial swelling and fibrinoid necrosis
	The hallmark skin findings are multiple well demarcated round or oval lesions that may have a lamellar crusting to the edge, akin to the rash of yaws
	Commonly reported in the pre-antibiotic era but there has been a resurgence of cases of lues maligna associated with HIV/AIDS
	Treatment of malignant syphilis may lead to a severe Jarisch–Herxheimer[c]
Latent syphilis	Asymptomatic (no evidence of primary, secondary, or tertiary disease) with positive serologic testing. Infection occurring within a year from exposure is considered early latent
	When latent infection is identified when exposure to diagnosis has been more than one year, it is considered late latent
Tertiary syphilis	Cardiac (within 10–30 years): thoracic aortic aneurysm, aortic regurgitation, and coronary artery ostial stenosis. All of these conditions are secondary to endarteritis (vasculitis of the *vasa vasorum*)
	Neurological
	1. Asymptomatic (less than 2 years from exposure)
	2. Acute syphilitic meningitis consisting of headache, meningeal irritation, confusion (5–7 years from exposure)
	3. Meningovascular with cranial nerve palsies[' d]
	4. General paresis (10–20 years from exposure) consisting of prodrome consisting of headache, vertigo, personality disturbances, followed by acute vascular event with focal findings
	5. Tabes dorsalis consisting of a clinical insidious onset of dementia associated with delusional state, fatigue, intention tremors, loss of facial-muscle tone, lightning pains, dysuria, ataxia, Argyll Robertson pupil, areflexia, loss of proprioception
	Gumma (1–46 years but most cases occur around 15 years from exposure) consisting of lesions presenting with monocytic infiltrates with associated tissue destruction of any organ

(Continued)

TABLE 9.9 Clinical Spectrum of Syphilis[a] (*cont.*)

Diseases	Core concepts
Neurosyphilis	Can occur at any stage of the natural history of syphilis Early neurological manifestations include isolated cranial nerve dysfunction, meningitis, stroke, uveitis, loss of vibration sense, or otitis media The diagnosis of neurosyphilis depends on a combination of cerebrospinal fluid (CSF) analysis including pleocytosis, elevated protein, and a reactive VDRL in CSF along with serologic evidence of syphilis and consistent neurologic syndrome. Among those with negative VDRL in CSF and in whom neurosyphilis is highly suspected, it is crucial obtaining and FTA–ABS testing on CSF[e] Late neurological manifestations of tertiary syphilis such as tabes dorsalis or general paresis occur 10–30 years after initial infection

[a]*A presumptive diagnosis of syphilis requires use of two serological tests: a nontrepnemal test (ie, VDRL—Venereal Disease Research Laboratory or RPR—Rapid Plasma Reagin which are nonspecific cardiolipin–cholesterol–lecithin regain antigen produced by the host in response to T. pallidum infection) and a treponemal test (ie, FTA-ABS—fluorescent treponemal antibody absorbed, TP-PA—T. pallidum passive particle agglutination, chemiluminescence immunoassays, immunoblots, or rapid treponemal assays). To diagnose a lesion exudate or tissue it is optimal to use darkfield examinations and tests to detect T. pallidum directly including PCR test (when available). False positive RPR can be due to antiphospholipid syndrome, systemic lupus erythematosus, pregnancy, tuberculosis, and other conditions).*

[b]*Frequently affects the posterior circulation (eg, Parinaud syndrome) and caused by two pathogenic forms: endarteritis obliterans of medium and large arteritis (ie, Heubner arteritis and Hissl–Alzheimer arteritis affecting small arterial vessels). Tends to occur about 5–7 years from initial exposure.*

[c]*Condyloma lata must be distinguished clinically from condyloma acuminatum caused by papillomavirus infection. Biopsy of perineal lesions shows plasma cell infiltrates associated with multiple treponemes using Warthin–Starry staining.*

[d]*The Jarisch–Herxheimer reaction is an acute febrile reaction frequently accompanied by headache, myalgia, fever, and other symptoms that can occur within the first 24 h after penicillin therapy. This reaction occurs more frequently during early infection due to higher treponemal burdens.*

[e]*Among persons with HIV infection, CSF leukocyte count is often elevated without neurosyphilis (>5 WBC/mm^3, so a cut-off of >20 WBC/mm^3 improves the specificity of neurosyphilis diagnosis.*

REFERENCES

1. Dembry LM, Andriole VT. Renal and perirenal abscesses. *Infect Dis Clin North Am* 1997;**11**(3):663–80.
2. Mody L, Juthani-Mehta M. Urinary tract infections in older women. A clinical review. *JAMA* 2014;**311**(8):844–54.
3. Ronald AR, Harding GKM. Complicated urinary tract infections. *Infect Dis Clin North Am* 1997;**11**(3):584–92.
4. Hammond NA, Nikolaidis P, Miller FH. Infectious and inflammatory diseases of the kidney. *Radiol Clin N Am* 2012;**50**:259–70.
5. Centers for Disease Control and Prevention. Sexually transmitted diseases treatment guidelines 2015. *MMWR* 2015;**64**(3):1–135.

Chapter 10

Cutaneous, Subcutaneous, and Deep Tissue Infections

DIAGNOSTIC APPROACH TO SKIN AND SOFT-TISSUE INFECTIOUS SYNDROMES

The Gram-positive bacteria *Streptococcus pyogenes* and *Staphylococcus aureus* represent the most important human pathogens that cause skin and soft-tissue infections.[1,2] Clostridial pathogens are also considered important infectious agents that may present with superficial cutaneous or deep tissue manifestations. Also, many Gram-negative bacterial pathogens, mycobacteria, parasitic, and fungi may cause severe life-threatening infections (Table 10.1). The clinical spectrum of skin and soft-tissue infections depends on the virulence of the infectious agent, production of toxins, and the host response to the infection.[1]

Group A streptococci (GAS) are classified by serotype based on the antigenically variable M surface protein (encoded by the *emm* gene). Although there are more than 200 types, serotype M1 is among the most frequently identified causing pharyngitis and invasive disease worldwide. This bacterium colonized epithelial surfaces of the oropharynx and skin. This colonization may transform into impetigo. However, GAS can also invade epitheliums and cause cellulitis, necrotizing fasciitis, bacteremia (Table 10.2), and streptococcal toxic shock syndrome (Table 10.3), it can also result in puerperal sepsis, meningitis, osteomyelitis, septic arthritis, pneumonia, and endocarditis. Group A streptococci adheres and invades epithelial cells and then enter the subepithelial tissue where neutrophils are recruited. Specific serotypes such as the M_1T_1 rapidly develops spontaneous mutations and resist neutrophil destruction allowing streptococci to promote tissue destruction by invading and producing tissue-disruptive exotoxins.

Occasionally pellagra caused by niacin deficiency may produce a well-demarcated eruption mimicking streptococcal cellulitis.

Similarly, *S. aureus* can not only produce impetigo but it may also invade sterile tissue and therefore cause invasive disease in the form of cellulitis, abscess, and impetigo. There are multiple other infectious agents associated with skin and soft-tissue infections that can be the result to exposure to animals or

Core Concepts in Clinical Infectious Diseases (CCCID). http://dx.doi.org/10.1016/B978-0-12-804423-0.00010-X

TABLE 10.1 Cutaneous Manifestations of Life-threatening Conditions

Pathogen	Disease	Core concepts
Neisseria meningitidis	Meningococcemia	Purpuric rash associated with septic shock Purpura fulminans (confluent petechial rash associated with coagulopathy)
Rickettsia ricketsii	Rocky Mountain spotted fever	Maculopapular rash associated with rapidly progressive disease
Ehrlichia chaffeensis *Ehrlichia ewingii*[a]	Human granulocytic ehrlichiosis	Maculopapular rash associated with rapidly progressive neurologic deterioration and respiratory failure in patients with HIV/AIDS
Capnocytophaga canomorsus *Streptococcus pneumoniae* *Haemophilus influenza* *Neisseria meningitidis*	Surgical removal of spleen or functional asplenia	Rapidly progressive sepsis. Patient may have purpuric rash or purpura fulminans or Waterhouse-Friderichsen Syndrome
S. aureus	Waterhouse–Friderichsen Syndrome	Reports in pediatric literature of this association with a purpuric rash and hemodynamic instability. This syndrome has also been associated with meningococcemia, disseminated histoplasmosis, tuberculosis, and other infectious diseases. Purpura fulminans which is characterized by the acute onset of progressive cutaneous hemorrhage and necrosis; and disseminated intravascular coagulation may occur during the Waterhouse–Friderichsen syndrome.
S. aureus *S. pyogenes*[b]	Toxic shock syndrome	Erythematous rash that becomes confluent and subsequently desquamates

TABLE 10.1 Cutaneous Manifestations of Life-threatening Conditions (*cont.*)

Pathogen	Disease	Core concepts
Drug reactions	Drug reaction eosinophilic systemic syndrome (DRESS)	Central maculopapular rash that becomes confluent associated with eosinophilia, elevated transaminases and bilirubin, and acute renal failure Associated to the administration of Vancomycin, ceftriaxone, or ciprofloxacin[c]
Other drug reactions	Toxic epidermal necrolysis (Lyell's syndrome)[d]	Can be related to the use of sulfa drugs, penicillin, cephalosporins Other drugs: allopurinol, NSAIDs, phenytoin
Acute bacterial endocarditis	*S. aureus*	Petechial rash, splinter hemorrhages and conjunctival petechiae
Erythema multiforme (EM)	Drug induced Infection associated: *Mycoplasma pneumoniae* or Herpes simplex-1 (HSV-1) or Herpes Simplex-2 (HSV-2), influenza B	Concomitant genital lesions or oral lesions may accompany HSV-1 or HSV-2 infections *Mycoplasma*-induced EM may occur concurrently with pneumonia or during convalescent phase
Protozoal	Free-living amoebas (infiltrative lesions of the skin may occur concomitantly with central nervous involvement)	*Balamuthia mandrilaris* *Acanthamoeba* *Sappinia*

[a]Paddock CD, Folk SM, Merril Shore G, Machado LJ, Huycke MM, Slater LN, et al. Infections with Ehrlichia chaffeensis *and* Ehrlichia ewingii *in persons coinfected with human immunodeficiency virus.* Clin Infect Dis 2001;**33**:1586–1594.
[b]Often associated with necrotizing fasciitis and S. pyogenes bacteremia.
[c]Jeung YJ, Lee JY, Oh MJ, Choi DC, Lee BJ. Comparison of the causes and clinical features of drug rash with eosinophilia and systemic symptoms and Stevens–Johnson syndrome allergy asthma. Immunol Res 2010;**2**(2):123–126.
[d]Stevens–Johnson syndrome is characterized by a less severe form, usually involving less than 10% of body surface area. TEN involves 30% or more of body surface area (Positive Nikolsky sign implies necrolysis).

TABLE 10.2 Clinical Spectrum of Skin and Soft-Tissue Infections

Category[a]	Etiologies	Core concepts
Impetigo	β-hemolytic streptococci and/or S. aureus Bullous impetigo is caused by strains of S. aureus that produce a toxin that causes cleavage of the granular layer of the epidermis (same toxin that causes Ritter's disease) Ecthyma is caused by impetigo lesions but ulcerations are deeper (ecthyma gangrenosum is a necrotic ulcerative lesion associated with Pseudomonas aeruginosa in patients with hematologic malignancies during episodes of neutropenia)	Associated with poor personal hygiene Bacteria initially colonized unbroken skin followed by their inoculation through skin abrasions, minor trauma, or insect bites Occurs most frequently in the face and extremities and bullae appear early with subsequent clear yellow fluid with thick crusts
Abscesses	Most frequently associated with S. aureus	Furuncles and carbuncles are most frequently caused by S. aureus
Cellulitis[b]	Cellulitis associated with furuncles, carbuncles, or abscesses is usually caused by S. aureus	In contrast, streptococci most commonly cause cellulitis not associated with a defined portal of entry.
	Cellulitis affects the upper dermis and subcutaneous fat	This is the most common form of cellulitis and more frequently associated with streptococci
	Periorbital cellulitis may be caused by Haemophilus influenzae, Streptococcus pneumoniae or Moraxella catarrhalis since this is often a result of acute bacterial sinusitis	Cellulitis and erysipelas are rapidly spreading areas of edema, erythema that sometimes is accompanied by lymphangitis and regional lymphadenopathy
	Cryptococcous may cause cellulitis among immunocompromised hosts	
Erysipelas	When the infectious process affects the upper dermis including the superficial lymphatics	The lesions are raised above the level of the surrounding skin and there is a clear demarcation between involved and involved tissue and associated with streptococci. Often the clinical distinction between cellulitis and erysipelas is challenging

TABLE 10.2 Clinical Spectrum of Skin and Soft-Tissue Infections (*cont.*)

Category[a]	Etiologies	Core concepts
Necrotizing fasciitis[c,d]	Type I (polymicrobial) Type II (usually *S. aureus*, *S. pyogenes*, or *Aeromonas hydrophila*) Characterized by widespread fascial necrosis with relative sparing of the underlying muscle when it is of polymicrobial origin In type II, there is usually myofasciitis with the potential complication of toxic shock syndrome Necrosis occurs due to thrombosis of fascial vasculature at all levels	The process initially begins the superficial fascial planes and progresses into deeper fascial layers causing necrosis by microvascular occlusion. The disease can be caused by *S. pyogenes, S. aureus, Vibrio vulnificus, Aeromonas hydrophila, and Edwardsiella tarda* (type II) or polymicrobial (type I). Fournier's gangrene is a type I process of the perineum. Type I is associated with peripheral vascular disease, diabetes mellitus, hematologic malignancies, postsurgical (posttransplantation), and chronic alcohol abuse
		Surgical management along with intravenous antibiotics and supportive care is crucial
Streptococcal toxic shock syndrome	No usual history of streptococcal pharyngitis Associated with necrotizing fasciitis Important association with Varicella–Zoster infection in children during chickenpox	Acute kidney injury manifests early in the course and the rash is not as prominent as in staphylococcal toxic shock syndrome. Localized muscle pain (more frequently identified during staphylococcal TSS)
Staphylococcal toxic shock syndrome	Menstrual Nowadays it is rarely seen but it was associated with the use of tampons	However many cases were due to use of sanitary pads regularly used during menstruation. Some of these cases are recurrent given persistent colonization with toxin producing bacteria
	Nonmenstrual	Surgical wound infections Influenza Skin and subcutaneous lesions including those caused by community-acquired skin and soft tissue infections (MRSA USA 300) Use of barrier contraceptives Nasal packing Postpartum Intravenous drug use[e] Frostbites Burns Use of NSAIDs

(Continued)

TABLE 10.2 Clinical Spectrum of Skin and Soft-Tissue Infections (*cont.*)

Category[a]	Etiologies	Core concepts
Clostridial myone-crosis (*C. perfringens, C. novyi, C. histolyticum, C. septicum*) (toxin-induced muscular necrosis and tissue injury and lecithinase-induced hemolysis)	Associated clinical conditions: Laparoscopic surgical procedures Musculoskeletal allografts Septic abortion Prolonged rupture of membranes and chorioamnionitis Presence of devitalized tissue caused by trauma, crush injury, enteric surgeries, biliary tract surgical procedures	Incubation period is usually within 48 h of event, but it can also in rare cases rarely weeks to manifest Gas-producing manifests as crepitus *C. perfringens* and *C. novyi* are increasingly reported among heroin users (black tar heroin) *C. septicum* is associated with individuals with hematologic ma-lignancies and during episodes of neutropenia or colon carcinomas Sometimes clostridial myonecrosis may rarely occur in some individuals without any predisposing risk factors Surgical management along with intravenous antibiotics and supportive care is crucial
Diabetic myone-crosis	Mechanism is likely due to muscle infarction due to arteriosclerosis obliterans	Presents as an acute onset of muscle pain, difficult ambulation (if located in the lower extremities) and no history of trauma. Treatment is supportive care and anti-inflammatory agents
Pyomyositis	Caused mainly by *S. aureus*	Affects individual muscle groups Rarely pyomyositis may be caused by *S. pneumoniae* or Gram-negative bacilli

[a]*Stevens DL, Bisno AL, Chambers HF, Everett ED, Dellinger P, Goldstein EJC, et al. Practice guidelines for the diagnosis and management of skin and soft-tissue infections.* Clin Infect Dis 2005;**41**:1373–1406.
[b]*Diseases or conditions that may masquerade as cellulitis include deep venous thrombosis, contact dermatitis, venous insufficiency associated dermatitis, gouty arthritis, Wells syndrome, Sweet's syndrome, erythromelalgia of myeloproliferative disorders, relapsing polychondritis, carcinoma erysipelatoides (inflammatory carcinomas –i.e., breast-), angioedema, Polyarteritis Nodosa, lipodermatosclerosis, morphea (scleroderma), lupus panniculitis, -1 antitrypsin deficiency panniculitis, cutaneous lymphoma, glucagonoma with necrolytic migratory erythema, leukemia cutis, chronic venous diseases (cutaneous necrotizing venous vasculitis, Mondor's disease (thrombophlebitis of breast tissue), superficial thrombophlebitis), and granulomatous mastitis (Falagas ME, Vergidis PI. Narrative review: diseases that masquerade as infectious cellulitis.* Ann Intern Med 2005;**142**:47–55; Wolinsky CD, Waldorf H. Chronic venous disease. Med Clin N Am 2009;**93**:1333–1346).
[c]*The diagnosis of necrotizing fasciitis is clinical but imaging studies may assist in the differential diagnosis. It is important to dissect the potential diseases that could resemble necrotizing fasciitis without the life-threatening consequences of this disease. In particular, it is important to consider paraneoplastic fasciitis as part of Sweet's syndrome, Schulman syndrome (eosinophilic fasciitis), nodular and proliferative fasciitis which is considered a benign pseudosarcomatous lesions, dermatomyositis, eosinophilic vasculitis with polyangiitis, lupus myofasciitis, graft-versus-host disease among those with a history of allogeneic transplantation, thymic transplantation, or blood transfusions, compartment syndrome and diabetic myonecrosis (Chaudry AA, Baker KS, Gould ES, Gupta R. Necrotizing fasciitis and its mimics: what radiologists need to know.* AJR 2015;**204**:128–139).
[d]*Umbert IJ, Winkelmann RK, Oliver FG, Peters MS. Necrotizing faciitis: A clinical, microbiologic, and histopathologic study of 14 patients.* J Am Acad Dermatol 1989;**20**:774–781.
[e]*Lowy FD, Gordon RJ. Bacterial infections in drug users.* N Engl J Med 2005;**353**(18):1945–1954.

TABLE 10.3 Clinical and Microbiological Criteria for Toxic Shock Syndrome

Category	Criteria
Streptococcal toxic shock syndrome[a]	
Pathogenic mechanism: Streptococcal pyrogenic exotoxin (SPE) and M protein. During invasive disease, M protein is shed and forms a complex with fibrinogen that then bind to the surface of polymorphonuclear leukocytes (PMNs). Once activated, PMNs release a wide variety of hydrolytic enzymes that damage the vascular endothelium causing vascular leakage and hypercoagulability resulting in hypotension, disseminated intravascular coagulation, and multiple organ injury[b]	Isolation of *S. pyogenes* from a normally sterile site or from a nonsterile site *Clinical signs of severity* Hypotension and; $\geq$ 2 of the following signs: Renal impairment Coagulopathy Liver function impairment Adult respiratory distress syndrome (ARDS)
Antitoxin used is intravenous immune globulin (IVIG)	A generalized erythematous maculopapular rash that desquamates Soft tissue necrosis, including necrotizing fasciitis, myositis, or gangrene
Staphylococcal toxic shock syndrome[c]	
Pathogenic mechanism: Toxic shock syndrome toxin-1 (TSST-1) act as a superantigen through its ability to bind Class II major histocompatibility complex of antigen-presenting cells and the Vβ region of the T-cell receptor stimulating an exuberant cytokine cascade from T-cell to hypotension and tissue injury No effective antitoxin (no evidence that IVIG improves outcomes)	A generalized erythematous maculopapular rash that desquamates Hypotension and; $\geq$ 2 of the following signs Renal impairment Coagulopathy Gastrointestinal Musculoskeletal (localized muscle pain) Liver function impairment

TSS, Toxic shock syndrome.
[a]*Patients with streptococcal toxin shock syndrome develops renal dysfunction early in the course. Most patients do not have evidence of active or recent streptococcal pharyngitis. Patients with staphylococccal TSS often have gastrointestinal symptomatology likely due to the action of TSST as enterotoxin or due to concomitant production of other staphylococci enterotoxins.*
[b]*Brown EJ. The molecular basis of streptococcal toxic shock syndrome. N Engl J Med 2004;**350**(20):2093–2094.*
[c]*S. aureus is identified in small fraction of cases, or isolated at a sterile site. Staphylococcal TSS is characterized by elevated fever, localized muscle pain, hypotension, and rash. The rash is often atypical to be considered as scarlet fever. Most cases are diagnosed based on clinical criteria as indicated in this table. The differential diagnosis of Staph TSS includes Strep TSS, meningococcemia, Kawasaki's disease, DRESS, rickettsial syndromes (rocky mountain spotted fever (RMSF) or human granulocytic ehrlichiosis), and scarlet fever.*

animal bites (Table 10.4); or exposure to waterborne pathogens (Table 10.5); and tick exposure[3] (Table 10.6). Additionally, a range of infectious or non-infectious diseases may manifest as nonhealing ulcers (Table 10.7), vesicles/blisters (Table 10.8), eschars or cutaneous necrosis (Table 10.9). Within the spectrum of clinical manifestations related with skin and soft-tissue infections, some of the systemic vasculitis that may involve skin and soft tissues (Table 10.10); exanthematous eruptions (Table 10.11); and urticarial lesions and angioedema of infectious origin or that are drug induced (Table 10.12).

Miscellaneous Skin and Soft Tissue Diseases

Infective Dermatitis

This entity was described in Jamaica and associated with recent infection by the human T-lymphotropic virus 1 (HTLV-1).[4] This condition is characterized by a chronic relapsing syndrome that usually affects young children presenting with generalized popular rash with exudates, and crusting on the scalp, ear, eyelid margins, neck, axilla, and groin. It can become secondarily impetiginized either by staphylococci or streptococci. In addition, individuals infected with HTLV-1 have an important association with crusted scabies (previously designated as Norwegian scabies) as well as disseminated strongyloidiasis.[4]

Hidradenitis Suppurativa

This is a primary dermatological condition that it is also known as "*acne inversa*." It is more frequent among African-American individuals. Hidradenitis suppurativa involves chronic inflammatory changes of the apocrine gland-bearing areas including the axilla, groin, and perianal region.[5] Men tend to more frequently develop perianal lesions whereas women tend to have involvement of the perineum. The disease initiates with discrete areas of dilated and occluded follicles and evolving into induration, scarring, pitting, and draining abscesses. It is crucial to recommend smoking cessation, weight loss; extreme hygiene of the affected areas, and in some situations long-term doxycycline is clinically useful. Surgical excision with roofing procedures is considered the only definitive therapy for severe cases. Drainage of secondarily infected glands and subcutaneous abscess may provide certain relief and, in some cases, promotes healing. Scarring of the affected areas may be severe and deforming.[5]

Exanthematous Eruptions

This group of eruptions (rashes) include those that are infectious and drug induced. Exanthematous drug eruptions are also called morbilliform or maculopapular drug eruptions. They are considered the most common forms of drug-induced eruptions. Other important drug-induced cutaneous manifestations (often systemic) include Stevens–Johnson syndrome (SJS)/toxic epidermic

TABLE 10.4 Infections Associated with Animal Exposure and Animal Bites

Pathogen	Disease	Core concepts
Francisella tularensis	Tularemia may also be tickborne (*Ixodes* spp) May also occur by handling infected animals, tick bites, or cat bites	It can occur in sheep handlers, wild game handling, pelt dealers, and veterinarians Spectrum of clinical forms: ulceroglandular, oculoglandular, glandular, oropharyngeal, typhoidal, and pneumonic syndromes
Pasteurella multocida or Canocytophaga canimorsus	Rapidly spreading cellulitis Animal bites may also cause septic arthritis, tendonitis, osteomyelitis, and subcutaneous abscesses	Dog bites or cat bites (*C. canimorsus* can cause rapidly progressive sepsis in asplenic individuals)
Streptobacillus moniliformis *Spirilus minus*	Rat bite fever[a]	*Streptobacillus* associated disease is characterized by abrupt onset of fever, arthritis, and rash that often involves palms and soles. Hemorrhagic vesicles may be seen (sometimes mimics disseminated gonococcal disease) *Spirillum* associated disease is insidious does not involve joints and sometimes causes by an ulcerated bite site and regional adenopathy. It is rare in the United States
HACEK group of organisms[a] Viridans-group streptococci	Human bites	Frequently associated with subcutaneous abscesses
Bartonella henselae	Cat scratch disease	Adenopathy Stellar retinitis Extranodal disease (spleen, liver, lung, bone, CNS) in 2% of cases
B. henselae *Bartonella quintana*	Bacillary angiomatosis	Among immunocompromised (eg, HIV/AIDS) with cutaneous lesions that resemble Kaposi's sarcoma

(Continued)

TABLE 10.4 Infections Associated with Animal Exposure and Animal Bites (*cont.*)

Pathogen	Disease	Core concepts
Yersinia pestis	Three clinical forms: septicemic, pneumonic and bubonic Bubonic is the most common and classic form develops when humans are bitten by infected fleas or have skin breach when handling contaminated animals or animal products Domestic cat scratches or bites may also transmit *Y. pestis*	Patient presents with fever, headache, chills, and ender regional lymphadenopathy a few days after exposure
Brucella mallei	Humans become infected through inhalation or skin contact	Pustular skin lesions and lymphadenopathy with suppurative adenopathy
Francisella tularensis	Ulceroglandular or glandular presentations	

[a]*HACEK organisms:* Haemophilus *species,* Aggregatibacter *species,* Cardiobacterium hominis, Eikenella corrodens, *and* Kingella *species.*

TABLE 10.5 Waterborne Pathogens Associated With Human Skin and Soft Tissue Infections[a]

Pathogen	Disease	Core concepts
Aeromonas hydrophila	Cellulitis, abscesses, bullae, or necrotizing fasciitis (more frequently seen than *Edwardsiella tarda*)	Fresh water exposure particularly estuary water. Most cases are due to traumatic inoculation
Vibrio vulnificus	Hemorrhagic bullae with associated sepsis May produce necrotizing fasciitis	Affects mostly individuals with chronic liver disease likely due to elevated iron levels
Edwardsiella tarda	Abscesses, bullae, myonecrosis, necrotizing fasciitis, cellulitis	Gram-negative rod that may secondarily infect wounds
Erysipelothrix rhusiopathiae	Localized violaceous cellulitis involving primarily hands or fingers in fish and meat handlers	Gram-positive rod whose major animal host is swine.

TABLE 10.5 Waterborne Pathogens Associated With Human Skin and Soft Tissue Infections[a] (*cont.*)

Pathogen	Disease	Core concepts
Mycobacterium marinum	Papular or nodular lympho-cutaneous lesions that develop in the extremities after trauma in fresh water, swimming pool, after handling seafood or associated with an aquarium	Exposure history should be carefully obtained
Streptococcus iniae	Cellulitis of the hand or digits	Percutaneous injuries occurring while handling fish (ie, fresh water fish such as tilapia)
Mycobacterium fortuitum	Furuncles	Fresh water exposure during pedicures

[a]*Janda JM, Abbott SL. The Genus Aeromonas: taxonomy, pathogenicity, and infection.* Clin Microb Rev *2010;23(1):35–73.*

TABLE 10.6 Tick borne Illnesses[a]

Category	Pathogen	Disease
Bacterial	*Borrelia*	Lyme disease
		Relapsing fever
	Rickettsia	Some examples:
		Human granulocytic ehrlichiosis
		(*E. chaffeensis, E. ewingii*)
		Anaplasmosis (*Anaplasma phagocytophilum*)
		Rocky Mountain spotted fever
		(RMSF)—*Rickettsia rickettsia*
	Spirochetes	Southern tick-associated rash illness (STARI) presumably caused by a spirochete carried by the tick *Amblyomma americanum* and resulting in a erythema migrans-like rash associated with a flu-like illness
	Francisella tularensis	Tularemia
Parasitic	*Babesia microti*	Babesiosis
Viral	Nairovirus	Crimean-Congo hemorrhagic fever
	Coltivirus	Colorado Tick-bite fever
	Flavivirus	Tick bite fever
		Powasan virus
	Bunyavirus	Severe fever and thrombocytopenia syndrome

[a]*With the only exception of* Borrelia duttonii *relapsing fever, tickborne illnesses that affect humans are zooanthroponoses (diseases of animals transmissible to humans where humans become incidental dead-end hosts). Ticks are second to mosquitoes in frequency of transmission of infectious diseases to humans.*

TABLE 10.7 Differential Diagnosis of Nonhealing Ulcers

Disease	Core concepts
Squamous cell carcinoma (verrucous)	Usually in the setting of longstanding inflammation
Pyoderma gangrenosum	Usually associated with rheumatoid arthritis, psoriatric arthritis, or inflammatory bowel disease
Nontuberculous mycobacteria	*Mycobacterium fortuitum* *Mycobacterium chelonei* *Mycobacterium abscessus*
Behcet's disease	Pathergy-associated lesions
Buruli ulcer	Infection caused by *Mycobacterium ulcerans*
Parasitic Bacterial Venous insufficiency Vascular insufficiency Pressure ulcers Neuropathic ulcers	Cutaneous leishmaniasis Mucocutaneous leishmaniasis Viscerotropic leishmaniasis (*L. tropica*) Melioidosis (*Burkholderia pseudomallei*) Chronic venous insufficiency ulcer Diabetic foot ulcers Decubitus ulcers Diabetes mellitus, leprosy (leprosy reactions), Dejerine–Sottas disease

TABLE 10.8 Clinical Spectrum of Diseases Manifesting as Vesicles/Blisters[a]

Condition	Core concepts
Large vessel or small-vessel Ischemia of the extremities	Blisters and bullae present in the affected areas
Streptococcal cellulitis or necrotizing fasciitis	Initial manifestation can be a blister with intense pain in the affected area and usually out of proportion to the clinical findings
Vibrio vulnificus	Hemorrhagic blisters and sepsis
Porphyria cutanea tarda	Hepatitis C is the most common cause Ethanol use/abuse
Contact dermatitis	Poison ivy Poison oak Neomycin (contained in topical antibiotic formulations)

TABLE 10.8 Clinical Spectrum of Diseases Manifesting as Vesicles/ Blisters (*cont.*)

Condition	Core concepts
Autoimmune	Bullous pemphigoid (tense blisters in older individuals with autoantibodies against the basement membrane)[b] Pemphigus vulgaris (autoimmune disease with autoantibodies against epidermal proteins causing acantholysis resulting in large, loose bullae, and patients tend to have oral mucosal involvement
Viral	Varicella–Zoster virus (chickenpox and herpes zoster) Rickettsialpox (*Rickettsia akari*) Monkeypox
Gluten intolerance	Dermatitis herpetiformis associated with gluten intolerance/celiac disease may mimic herpes zoster
Porphyria cutanea tarda	Associated with chronic viral hepatitis C and also associated with chronic alcohol abuse
Neutrophilic dermatoses	Pyoderma gangrenosum may manifest with a bullous configuration Sweet's syndrome has been associated with hemorrhagic blisters
Linear IgA bullous dermatosis (LABD)	Characterized by symmetrically distributed, tense, sausage-like bullae or vesicles in strikingly annular or polycyclic plaques ("string of pearls" or "crown of jewels").[c] It has been associated with the administration of penicillins, cephalosporins, and vancomycin. Also associated with inflammatory bowel disease and with some malignancies

[a]*Tzanck smear is clinically useful in selected situations in the diagnostic workup of vesculobullous diseases(Kelly B, Shimoni T. Reintroducing the Tzanck smear. Am J Clin Dermatol 2009;**10**(3): 141–142).*
[b]*Necrolysis is present in toxic epidermal necrolysis (TEN) and staphylococcal scalded skin syndrome but absent in bullous pemphigoid. Epidermolysis bullosa is caused by autoantibodies against the basement membrane (collagen type VII) and causes blisters usually after trauma.*
[c]*Johnson EF, Jacobs MH, Smidt AC. Annular vesiculobullous eruption in a healthy young man. JAMA 2013;**310**(23):2559–2560.*

TABLE 10.9 Differential Diagnosis of Cutaneous Eschars or Necrotic Lesions[a]

Bacterial	Cutaneous anthrax (*Bacillus anthracis*)	Usually not associated with systemic forms of the disease (mediastinal form associated with septic shock)
	Chromobacterium violaceum	Seen in patients with chronic granulomatous disease
	Pseudomonas aeruginosa	Ecthyma gangrenosum
	Treponema pallidum	Secondary syphilis, malignant syphilis (Lues maligna)
	Erysipelothrix rhusiopathiae	Violaceous cellulitic process in hands and digits among fish and meat handlers
	Mycobacterial	Cutaneous tuberculosis (tuberculosis verrucosa cutis)
		Mycobacterium fortuitum/*M. chelonei* associated with subcutaneous administration of aesthetic contaminated products
		Lucio's phenomenon in Diffuse Lepromatous Leprosy of Lucio (occurs mostly in patients from Mexico, Central America, and Iranian individuals)
	Lyme's disease	Erythema migrans may become necrotic
	Plague (*Yersinia pestis*)	Necrotic area at site of entry with associated with adenopathy
	Tularemia (*Francisella tularensis*)	Necrotic area at site of entry with associated with adenopathy
Calciphylaxis	Calcyphic uremic arteriolopathy	Non-uremic: Malignancy (ovarian carcinoma, melanoma, Hodgkin's disease) Autoimmune (Scleroderma Polymyositis, Dermatomyositis)
Neutrophilic dermatoses	Pyoderma gangrenosum Sweet's syndrome	Inflammatory Bowel Disease Rheumatoid arthritis psoriatric arthritis
Fungal	Mucormycosis (*Absidia Cunninghamella Rhizopus*)	Also sporotrichosis may produce necrotic lesions
	Phaeophymycosis (Dermatocius fungi) *Exophialia Bipolaris*	Chromoblastomycosis (*Fonseca pedrosoi*)
Coumadin necrosis	Patients with Protein C or Protein S deficiency maybe at the highest risk	Necrosis tends to occur in fat areas

TABLE 10.9 Differential Diagnosis of Cutaneous Eschars or Necrotic Lesions[a] (*cont.*)

Bites of brown recluse spiders (*Loxosceles reclusa*)[b]	Brown recluse spider	Necrotic arachnidism
Cryoglobulinemia	Hepatitis C associated	Large areas of cutaneous eschars/ necrosis
Diabetic	Diabetic ulcer	Areas of necrosis
Necrotizing vasculitis	Leukocytoclastic vasculitis Polyarteritis nodosa Takayasu's	
Tick-borne	Spotted fever rickettsias	*Rickettsia africae* *Rickettsia parker* Murine typhus
Parasitic infections	Leishmaniasis	Mucocutaneous leishmaniasis Viscerotropic leishmaniasis (*L. tropica*)
Vascular occlusive or venous disease	Antiphospholipid syndrome Arterial disease Venous stasis ulcers Livedoid vasculopathy Small-vessel occlusive	Ischemic limb gangrene with palpable pulses (produces two distinct syndromes: venous limb gangrene—early disease is called phlegmasia cerluea dolens—and symmetric peripheral gangrene)[c]
Malignancy associated	Mycosis fungoides Basal cell carcinomas Squamous cell carcinomas Malignant melanomas Leukemia cutis Lymphomatoid papulosis	Papulonecrotic disease
Immobility	Pressure ulcers	Insufficient tissue oxygenation

[a]*Swanson DL, Vetter RS. Bites of brown recluse spiders and suspected necrotic arachnidism. N Engl J Med 2005;352:700–707.*
[b]*Bites of venomous snakes may also produce localized tissue necrosis (Gold BS, Dart RC, Barish RA. Bites of venomous snakes. N Engl J Med 2002;347(5):347–355).*
[c]*Symmetric peripheral gangrene is associated with septic shock (e.g., meningococcemia) or cardiogenic shock while venous limb gangrene is associated with heparin-induced thrombocytopenia, paraneoplastic from adenocarcinomas, and antiphospholipid syndrome (Warketin TE. Ischemic limb gangrene with pulses. N Engl J Med 2015;373(7):642–655).*

TABLE 10.10 Clinical Approach to Systemic Vasculitis with Cutaneous Involvement

Category of vasculitis	Disease	Core concepts
Small-vessel or medium size vessel vasculitis	Lupus vasculitis	Low or normal complement levels. Association with Systemic Lupus or subacute cutaneous lupus. Acral lesions lasting more than 24 h[a]
	Polyarteritis nodosa	Nodular lesions, livedo reticularis. Associated with hepatitis B infection
	Granulomatous polyangiitis	Respiratory and renal involvement, gingival hyperplasia
	Cryoglobulinemic vasculitis	Elevated rheumatoid factor and associated with chronic hepatitis C infection. Acral lesions, peripheral neuropathy, decreased C4 levels, triad of purpura, arthralgia, and weakness and overlaps with Sjögren syndrome
	Henoch-Schönlein Purpura (HSP)	After an upper respiratory infection (*S. pyogenes*). Most common cause of leukocytoclastic vasculitis in children[b]. Association with *Helicobacter pylori*. Associated with acute hemorrhagic edema of infancy
Small-vessel vasculitis	Drug-induced hypersensitivity vasculitis	Drugs: propylthiouracil, penicillins, cephalosporins, sulfa drugs, isotretinoin, hydralazine. There has been an increasing recognition of proton-pump-inhibitors, particularly pantoprazole inducing subcutaneous lupus erythematosus
	Urticarial vasculitis	Low or normal complement levels, angioedema, association with hematologic malignancies, fever, uveitis, arthritis, pulmonary and renal disease

[a]*In direct immunofluorescence assay there is C3, IgG, and IgM perivascular deposition in basement-membrane zone in urticarial vasculitis, lupus vasculitis, polyarteritis nodosa, and granulomatous angiitis. In cryoglobulinemia there is perivascular IgM deposition, whereas in HSP there is perivascular IgA, and in hypersensitivity vasculitis there is fibrin and C3 deposition.*
[b]*The term leukocytoclastic refers to the debris of polymorphonuclear cells within the blood vessel walls associated with small vessel vasculitis.*

TABLE 10.11 Differential Diagnosis of Exanthematous Eruptions

Etiology	Core concepts
Exanthematous drug eruption[a]	Most frequent drug-induced reactions to medications. Topical steroids are helpful. Severe reactions may have mucosal involvement and fever. Eruption is coalescent pink-to-red maculopapular usually in the thorax and back
Measles	Morbilliform rash, sometimes itchy, and often blanching erythematous macules. Rash begins in the head and neck and spreads rapidly. Koplik's spots on the buccal mucosa and conjunctivitis.
Rubella	Similar rash to measles but rash improves within a few days (4–5 days). There is fever, adenopathy (occipital), and arthralgias
Erythema infectiosum (fifth disease caused by Parvovirus B19)[b]	Young children with slapped cheeks, fever develops 2–4 days prior to diffuse rash, which starts on proximal extremities and spreads both centrally and peripherally. Adults experience arthralgias/arthritis. The rash follows a livedo pattern and facial involvement is rare in adults
Roseola infantum (HHV-6 or HHV-7)	Sometimes fever may last for many weeks in adults. The rash usually starts in the trunk and spreads to face and extremities. Children start with high fevers for 3 to 5 days followed by a rash that is pink and short-lived.
Enterovirus (Echo, Coxsackie)	During summer months and sometimes occurring along with meningitis and gastrointestinal symptoms
Infectious Mononucleosis and mononucleosis like-illness associated early HIV-infection	Epstein-Barr virus may induce an exanthematous rash when active disease is present and antibiotics, usually beta-lactams produce a characteristic exanthematous eruption
Graft-versus-host disease	Symmetric exanthematous rash with lymphadenopathy, pharyngitis, arthralgias sometimes involving face, palms, and soles Characteristically occurs 2–4 weeks from transplantation and mimics an exanthematous drug eruption
Dengue virus	Morbilliform sandpaper-like on the trunk (rash is much less frequent with other flaviviruses such as West Nile Virus); also rare with togaviruses such as chikungunya

[a]*Stern RS. Exantematous drug eruptions. N Engl J Med 2012;366:2492–2501.*
[b]*Classification of viral diseases according to their description: first disease (measles); second disease (scarlet fever); third disease (rubella); fourth disease (Dukes' disease which may not exist but others believe it is Ritter's disease or staphylococcal scalded skin syndrome); fifth disease (erythema infectiousum caused by Parvovirus B19); and sixth disease (roseola infantum or roseola subitum associated with human herpes virus-6 HHV-6 or HHV-7). Enteric fever, specifically, when caused by Salmonella Typhi may have rose spots which are blanching papules usually found on the trunk.*

TABLE 10.12 Infectious Causes of Urticarial Lesions and Selected Causes of Angioedema[a]

Urticaria	Angioedema
Fasciola hepatica Visceral larva migrans (*Toxocara cati/ Toxocara canis*) Acute hepatitis B	*Infectious* Filarial (*Loa loa* causing calabar swellings) Sulfa drugs, beta-lactam drugs Dental abscesses may trigger angioedema in susceptible individuals (ie, those with hereditary angioedema)
Strongyloides stercolaris, Ancylostoma duodenale, Necator americanus *Trichinella spiralis* Enterovirus (Coxsackie, echo) *Mycoplasma pneumonia*	*Hereditary* Type 1 deficiency of C1 esterase inhibitor Type 2 dysfunction of C1 esterase inhibitor Type 3 associated with mutation of Factor XII
Cercarial dermatitis (acute schistosomiasis, also termed swimmers' itch)	*Acquired* Type 1: Lymphoproliferative disorders Type 2: Autoimmune with secondary development of antibodies against C1 esterase inhibitor *Medication induced* (Angiotensin converting enzyme inhibitors) *Physically induced* (cold, heat, vibration, trauma, emotional stress, ultraviolet light) *Cytokine-dysfunction* (Gleich's syndrome) Thryoid autoimmune disease

[a]Temino VM, Peebles S Jr. *The spectrum and treatment of angioedema.* Am J Med 2008;**121**:282–286.

necrolysis (TEN), acute generalized exanthematous pustulosis (AGEP), and drug reaction with eosinophilia and systemic symptoms (DRESS). These drug eruptions are idiosyncratic, T-cell-mediated delayed type IV hypersensitivity reactions. Exanthematous drug eruptions are often pruritic that appear 4–21 days after an individual initiates the eliciting medication. The rash is usually symmetrically distributed and characterized by pink-to-red macules and papules that coalesce and spread rapidly and must be distinguished from other exanthematous eruptions not related to medications (Table 10.11). Finally, urticarial, fixed drug eruptions (red round plaques that sting resulting in long-term pigmentation of the affected area and usually caused by nonsteroidal antiinflammatory drugs (NSAIDs), beta-lactam drugs, sulfa drugs and acetaminophen), and photosensitivity account for the rest of drug-associated cutaneous diseases. Urticaria and angioedema are frequently drug-induced and caused by NSAIDs or by angiotensin-converting-enzyme inhibitors. Nonetheless, there are infectious diseases that need to be considered associated with urticarial or angioedema (Table 10.12). Photosensitivity reactions are mainly caused by tetracyclines, voriconazole, and quinolones.

Mycetomas

These conditions encompass a group of chronic subcutaneous inflammatory granulomatous infectious processes that are divided in two types: eumycetomas or *true mycetoma* caused by fungi and actinomycetoma caused by aerobic filamentous bacteria. Actinomycetomas are caused by members of the genera *Nocardia, Streptomyces, Nocardiopsis*, and *Actinomadura*. Fungal mycetomas are most frequently caused by members of the genera *Madurella and Acemonium*. Of these, *Madurella mycetomatis* is the most prevalent causative pathogen. The term mycetoma coined by Vandyke Carter in 1860, suggests a fungal tumor; however, aerobic filamentous bacteria cause most cases worldwide (60% of cases). Mycetomas are also frequently identified as *Madura foot*.[6]

Botryomycosis

This is a chronic, purulent and granulomatous bacterial infection usually involving the skin and subcutaneous tissue.[7] *S. aureus* is usually the pathogen causing botryomycosis in more than 40% of cases followed by *Pseudomonas aeruginosa* and less frequently by coagulase-negative staphylococci *a* and other bacterial pathogens. Factors involved in its occurrence include an intermediate inoculum of the bacteria and the immunologic status of the host. The Splendore-Hoeppli phenomenon involves the formation of grains and is characteristic of this condition. Most clinical presentations produce nodularlike and suppurative lesions but there are visceral forms of botryomycosis. The differential diagnosis includes mycetoma, actinomycosis, cutaneous tuberculosis, and epidermal cysts and abscesses.

REFERENCES

1   Cole JN, Barnett TC, Nizet V, Walker MJ. Molecular insight into invasive group A streptococcal disease. *Nature Rev Microbiol* 2011;**9**:724–36.
2   Daum RS. Skin and soft-tissue infections caused by Methicillin-resistant *Staphylococcus aureus*. *N Engl J Med* 2007;**357**(4):380–90.
3   Parola P, Raoult D. Ticks and tickborne bacterial diseases in humans: an emerging infectious threat. *Clin Infect Dis* 2001;**32**:897–928.
4   Verdonck K, Gonzalez E, Van Dooren S, Vandamme AM, Vanham G, Gotuzzo E. Human T-lymphotropic virus 1 recent knowledge about an ancient infection. *Lancet Infect Dis* 2007;**7**:266–81.
5   Shah N. Hidradenitis suppurativa: a treatment challenge. *Am Fam Physician* 2005;**72**:1547–54.
6   Tellez I, Franco-Paredes C. A woman with subcutaneous swelling of the right foot associated with sinus tracts discharging yellowish grains. *PLoS Negl Trop Dis* 2010;**4**(9):e772.
7   Bonifaz A, Carrasco E. Botryomycosis. *Int J Dermatol* 1996;**35**(6):381–7.

Chapter 11

Osteoarticular Infections

DIAGNOSTIC APPROACH TO OSTEOARTICULAR INFECTIONS

Monoarthritis and Polyarthritis

Compared to the symptom of "*arthralgia*," which is pain of a joint or multiple joints without associated synovitis, the term "*arthritis*" is associated with the cardinal signs and symptoms of inflammation: swelling, erythema, and pain associated with synovitis. The differential diagnosis of monoarthritis (oligoarthritis) is different (Table 11.1) than the differential of a patient presenting with multiple joints involved (polyarthritis) (Table 11.2). Joint involvement may be simultaneous, additive, or migratory. Some individuals may present with migratory inflammation of the joints (Table 11.3). Some clinically useful pointers associated with polyarthritis include the following:

- Bacteria may be identified on Gram's-staining of synovial fluid in 50–75% of cases and culture in more than 90% of cases in the absence of antimicrobial therapy prior to obtaining cultures
- In a minority of patients, there is juxtaarticular osteomyelitis and effusions which may require surgical debridement or percutaneous aspiration
- Septic joints may not always be red, warm, and extremely painful
- Pain disproportionately greater than joint effusion may occur in rheumatic fever, familial Mediterranean fever (FMF), acute leukemia, and in patients with HIV/AIDS
- Rheumatoid factor may not only be reactive in rheumatoid arthritis but also in viral arthritis, bacterial endocarditis, sarcoidosis, and tuberculosis-related Poncet's reactive arthritis
- Some conditions may present with episodic recurrences: Lyme disease, crystal-induced arthropathies (gout and pseudogout), Whipple's disease, familial Mediterranean fever, adult-onset Still's disease (AOSD), systemic lupus erythematosus, inflammatory bowel disease, and sarcoidosis
- Systemic leucocytosis is not exclusive of septic arthritis. It may occur with Still's disease, acute leukemia, and systemic vasculitis
- Synovial fluid is essential in establishing a specific diagnosis, particularly when suspecting septic arthritis, reactive arthritis or inflammatory arthritis (ie, crystal-induced arthropathies) (Table 11.4).

Core Concepts in Clinical Infectious Diseases (CCCID). http://dx.doi.org/10.1016/B978-0-12-804423-0.00011-1

TABLE 11.1 Differential Diagnosis of Acute Monoarthritis[a]

Category	Etiology	Core concepts
Infectious	Bacteria	S. aureus, Streptococcus pyogenes, Streptococcus pneumoniae, Streptococcus agalactiae, Haemophilus influenza, Escherichia coli. Neisseria gonorrhoeae, Salmonella spp., Neisseria meningitidis
	Mycobacteria	Mycobacterium tuberculosis, Mycobacterium kansasii
	Lyme disease	B. burdorgferi
	Viral	Chikungunya, HIV, Rubella
Inflammatory	Osteoarthritis	Cartilage destruction
Trauma	Fracture Internal derangement	Sometimes fat droplets identified in fluid analysis
Crystal related	Gout (monosodium urate crystals)	Sometimes presence of tophi
	Pseudogout (calcium pyrophosphate dehydrate crystals)	May have evidence of chondrocalcinosis on radiograph images. Pseudogout may provide first clue to hyperparathyroidism, acromegaly, hemochromatosis, or hypomagnesemia
	Apatite crystals	Apatite-related arthropathy (periarthritis/tendinitis usually in the shoulder with calcific changes; Milwaukee shoulder syndrome with a history of trauma or overuse of the joint; osteoarthritis, erosive arthritis)
	Calcium oxalate crystals	Associated with end-stage renal disease and hemodialysis; short bowel syndrome, thiamine or pyridoxine deficiency; diets rich in rhubarb, spinach or ascorbic acid; primary oxalosis
Neoplastic	Pigmented villonodular synovitis Metastasis Osteoid osteoma	
Hematologic	Hemophilia Anticoagulation Sickle cell disease	Hemarthrosis Hemarthrosis Vasoocclusive phenomena

TABLE 11.1 Differential Diagnosis of Acute Monoarthritis (*cont.*)

Category	Etiology	Core concepts
Systemic autoinflammatory or autoimmune diseases	Psoriatric arthritis Behcet's disease Systemic lupus erythematosus Sarcoidosis Inflammatory bowel disease Reactive arthritis	May present with monoarticular disease May have a history of pathergy, recurrent oral and genital ulcers May cause oligoarthritis of large-joints with fever and sometimes it is confused with disseminated gonococcal infection May have concurrent rash, diarrhea, urethritis, or uveitis
Prosthetic joint	Prosthetic joint infection Aseptic loosening	Occult or overt bacteremia leading to secondary seeding. Often, if coagulase negative staphylococci involved, infection may have been acquired at the time of arthroplasty

ªBaker DG, Schumacher HR. Acute monoarthritis. N Engl J Med *1993;**329**(14):1013–1019.*

Septic Arthritis

Infection of a joint is a true medical emergency requiring early institution of antibiotics and joint drainage (percutaneous or surgical). *Staphylococcus aureus* and Group A, Group B, Group C, and Group G *Streptococcus* are becoming the most important etiologies of septic arthritis (Table 11.1). The incidence of disseminated gonococcal disease with joint involvement continues to be also a concern, but certainly, not as often as described before the antibiotic era. Septic arthritis is most often the result of occult bacteremia and given the fact that the synovium is a highly vascular structure that lacks a protective basement membrane, it becomes vulnerable to secondary bloodstream infectious seeding. Articular damage in septic arthritis results not only from multiple factors, such as tissue ischemia, bacterial invasion eliciting a strong inflammatory response but also due to bacterial enzymes or toxins entering the joint. Since cartilage is avascular and highly dependent on its nourishment by the synovium, joint pressure increase along with purulent exudates affects blood flow leading to cartilage anoxia. Gram-positive organisms express molecular receptors that attach to collagen, laminin, fibronectin, and other macromolecules of the articular matrix. The most important risk factor for septic arthritis is preexisting articular disease leading to expression of potential molecular receptors capable of facilitating secondary seeding during an episode of bloodstream infection.

TABLE 11.2 Differential Diagnosis of Polyarthritis[a]

Category	Associated conditions
Autoimmune	Rheumatoid arthritis Adult onset Still's disease Psoriatic arthritis Systemic lupus erythematosus (Jaccoud's arthropathy) Systemic vasculitis
Infectious	Bacterial septic arthritis Bacterial endocarditis[b] Lyme disease Mycobacterial Fungal Viral arthritis
Reactive (postinfectious)	Bacterial (enterocolitis or sexually transmitted) Viral (chikungunya, parvovirus B19) Mycobacterial (pulmonary tuberculosis causing Poncet's disease)
Miscellaneous	Familial Mediterranean fever Sarcoidosis Kawasaki's disease Erythema nodosum Erythema multiforme Pyoderma gangrenosum Dermatomyositis Henoch–Schönlein purpura Behcet's disease
Inflammatory	Crystal-induced (gout or pseudogout)

[a]*Pinals RS. Polyarthritis and fever. N Engl J Med 1994;**330**(11):769–774.*
[b]*Endocarditis manifests in many cases with lower back pain, but approximately 10–15% may present with one to three joints inflammed during an acute episode of endocarditis without evidence of bacteria when joints were aspirated in many cases (Pinals RS. Polyarthritis and fever. N Engl J Med 1994;**330**(11):769–774). Therefore, clinicians need to consider fever with lower back pain in the differential diagnosis of acute bacterial endocarditis.*

Reactive Arthritis

In some individuals, after an episode of enteritis/gastroenteritis/enterocolitis caused by either *Salmonella, Shigella, Campylobacter*, or *Yersinia* may result in an asymmetric additive polyarthritis involving predominantly the large joints in lower extremities. Similarly urogenital infection (sexually acquired) caused mainly by *Chlamydia trachomatis* may lead to the same manifestations. A minority of patients with arthritis associated with genital infections have the triad of conjunctivitis, urethritis, and arthritis (previously Reiter's syndrome) (Tables 11.2 and 11.3). Most individuals share the HLA-B27 as an identifiable marker of predisposition. Yersiniosis may manifest with pharyngitis, cervical

TABLE 11.3 Differential Diagnosis of Migratory Polyarthritis[a]

Category	Etiology	Core concepts
Infectious bacterial	*Neisseria gonorrhoea*	Disseminated gonococcal infection frequently results in petechial or pustular acral skin lesions, asymmetric polyarthralgia, tenosynovitis or oligoarticular or polyarticular septic arthritis.[b] Only 10–20% of adult experience polyarticular involvement affecting large joints
	Lyme's disease	Usually monoarticular but rarely may be polyarticular
	S. aureus *Tropheryma whippelli*	Can produce monoarticular or polyarticular Whipple's disease
Infectious viral	Arthropod transmitted alpha-viruses (ie, chikungunya)[c,d]	Oceania [Barmah Forest virus (BFV) and Ross River viruses (RRV)] Africa (O'nyong-nyong Virus (ONNV), Semliki Forest virus (SFV) South America (Mayaro) Africa, Asia, Scandinavia, Russia (Sindbis virus (SINV) and Sindbis-like viruses
Other viral	Hepatitis B (preceding hepatitis phase) Rubella Parvovirus B19 HIV	HIV (septic arthritis, reactive, or seronegative spondyloarthropathies)
Inflammatory	Reactive arthritis (postinfectious)	Posturethritis (ie, Chlamydia) Postgastrointestinal (ie, Shigellosis) Rheumatic fever Poststreptococcal arthritis caused by *Streptococcus pyogenes* (not meeting criteria for rheumatic fever) Poncet's disease[e] (pulmonary or extrapulmonary tuberculosis). In this setting, arthritis needs to be distinguished from pyrazinamide induced hyperuricermia and gout
	Crystalline arthropathies	Gout or pseudogout in adult patients usually with established diagnosis of crystal-induced disease
	Inflammatory bowel disease	About 10–20% may have polyarthritis. Inflammatory bowel disease, Whipple's disease may have to be distinguished by intestinal/colonic biopsies and associated clinical picture

(Continued)

TABLE 11.3 Differential Diagnosis of Migratory Polyarthritis (*cont.*)

Category	Etiology	Core concepts
Autoimmune	Rheumatic fever (*Streptococcus pyogenes*)	Jaccoud's arthropathy (see subsequently)
	Systemic lupus Erythematosus (SLE)	Patients with SLE may experience polyarthralgias in more than 95% of cases. Jaccoud's arthropathy may occur in SLE with reducible deformities and resulting mainly from soft-tissue abnormalities such as laxity of ligaments, fibrosis of the capsule, and muscular imbalance, rather than from destruction of the bone of joints, as it occurs in rheumatoid arthritis
	Granulomatous polyangiitis (Wegener's granulomatosis)	May initially manifest as fever and polyarthritis prior to pulmonary and renal manifestations
Neoplastic	Acute leukemia	Acute lymphoblastic leukemia Acute myelocytic leukemias

[a]*Pinals RS. Polyarthritis and fever. N Engl J Med 1994;**330**(11):769–774; Casey JD, Solomon D, Gaziano TA, Miller AL, Loscalzo J. A patient with migrating polyarthritis. N Engl J Med 2013;**369**:75–80.*
[b]*Disseminated gonococcal infection may cause the following manifestations: arthritis, arthritis-dermatitis syndrome (acral pustular skin lesions with tenosynovitis and septic arthritis), perihepatitis (Fitz–Hugh–Curtis syndrome), right-sided endocarditis, meningitis.*
[c]*Caglioti C, Lalle E, Castilletti C, Carletti F, Capobianchi MR, Bordi L. Chikungunya virus infection: an overview. New Microbiologica 2013;**36**:211–227.*
[d]*Chikungunya derives its name from Makonde, a language spoken in South Tanzania meaning: that which bends up referring to the posture of patients afflicted with severe arthralgias associated with this viral infection. Most patients developed systemic affection with myocarditis, meningoencephalitis, but often retinitis.*
[e]*Franco-Paredes C, Diaz-Borjon A, Barragán L, Senger M, Leonard M. The ever-expanding association between tuberculosis and rheumatologic diseases. Am J Med 2006;**119**:470–477.*

adenopathy and arthritis leading to confusion with *Streptococcus pyogenes* causing rheumatic fever or *Streptococcus* associated reactive arthritis. Symptoms may begin with entesophathy (pain tendon insertion site), dactylitis (sausage digits) followed by large joint affection and most commonly occurring 1 or 2 weeks after the initial enterocolitic or urogenital clinical presentation.

Some patients may experience postviral reactive arthritis. The most relevant viral pathogen that induced a long-term postinfectious syndrome is chikungunya with severe arthralgias in many patients; and often synovitis in a minority of cases. Other alpha-viruses (togaviruses) may produce a postinfectious arthritis/arthralgia syndrome (Tables 11.2 and 11.3). There are also other cases of reactive arthritis associated with dengue or other flaviviruses.

TABLE 11.4 Differential Diagnosis of Synovial Fluid Analysis[a]

Category	Etiology	Core concepts[b]
Healthy	Normal synovial fluid	Fewer than 180 cells per cubic millimeter with mononuclear predominance
Noninflammatory (<2000 cells per cubic millimeter)	Osteoarthritis	Fewer than 2000 cells per cubic millimeter with mononuclear predominance
Inflammatory (2,000–50,000 cells per cubic millimeter)	Crystal induced	More than 2000 cells per mm³ to 50,00. Pseudogout may have a particularly elevated white blood cell count in synovial fluid analysis
	Rheumatoid arthritis or seronegative arthritis	May present with 2,000–20,000 white blood cells (WBC) per cubic millimeter. Some patients present with "pseudosepsis" which consists of acute synovitis, fever, leucocytosis, high-WBC in synovial fluid and culture-negative, purulent synovial effusions that improve without antibiotic therapy[c]
Infectious (>50,000 cells per cubic millimeter)	Bacterial	More than 100,000 cells per mm³ with PMN predominance is highly suggestive of infection[d] particularly if the Gram stain and/or culture demonstrates presence of bacteria[e]

[a]Baker DG, Schumacher HR. Acute monoarthritis. N Engl J Med 1993;**329**(14):1013–1019.
[b]Fluid should be analyzed for cell counts, Gram-stain and culture, and search for crystals, fat droplets (fracture and trauma), and when indicated molecular testing (PCR) for Borrelia burdorgferi to confirm a diagnosis of Lyme's arthritis.
[c]Fuchs HA. Polyarticular pseudosepsis in rheumatoid arthritis. South Med J 1992;**85**:381–383.
[d]A patient may have less than 100,000 cells per cubic millimeter and still may have septic arthritis. The presence of crystals does not exclude infection, since a history of gout may predispose patients to septic arthritis. Some patients require synovial biopsy and arthroscopy.
[e]Synovial white blood cell counts (WBC) may be helpful in suspecting or confirming the possibility of septic arthritis. However, a finding of elevated polymorphonuclears (PMN > 90%) is useful in assessing the possibility of septic arthritis. An elevated WBC in synovial fluid, usually above 50,000 per cubic millimeter associated with more than 90% PMN highly suggests septic arthritis (Margaretten ME, Kohlwess J, Moore D, Bent S. Does this adult patient have septic arthritis? JAMA 2007;**297**(13):1478–1488; Ross JJ. Septic arthritis. Infect Dis Clin N Am 2005;**19**:799–817).

Septic Bursitis

This condition refers to inflammation caused by an infectious agent of a bursa, which are sac-like structures that protect soft tissues from underlying bony prominences. Septic bursitis results from direct inoculation due to trauma, spread of a nearby cellulitis or abscess, or due to hematogenous spread (bloodstream infection).[1] There are more than 100 bursae in the human body in both superficial (subcutaneous) and deep tissues (around tendons inserting into bones) and they contain some synovial fluid producing synovial cells. In addition to infectious causes of bursitis, these structures may become inflamed due to trauma, crystal-induced inflammation, or associated with systemic disorders. Risk factors for septic bursitis include diabetes mellitus, alcohol abuse, rheumatoid arthritis, and tophaceous gout. Clinical diagnosis is important since confusion with septic arthritis may lead to inadvertent inoculation of an infectious pathogen intraarticularly through a diagnostic arthrocentesis. A useful clinical distinction is that with septic bursitis most patients are still able to flex the extremity, whereas with septic arthritis, most patients have exquisite pain during flexion. Most common pathogens include *S. aureus* and streptococci (group A, B, C, or G). Management requires intravenous antibiotics and percutaneous or surgical drainage of infected fluid. The knee is the most frequently involved joint due to bacterial septic arthritis with polyarticular involvement seen in 10–20% of cases with an average of affection of four joints. Most frequent bacterial causes of septic polyarthritis include gonococcal, pneumococcal, Group B streptococci, and Gram-negative bacilli.

Prosthetic Joint Infections

Similar to other prosthetic devices, biofilm development associated with particular bacterial pathogens plays a crucial role in the pathogenesis of prosthetic joint infections. In many settings, with an increasing number of prosthetic joint replacement surgeries, there has been a concomitant increase in infections associated to these prosthetic devices. Risk factors for prosthetic joint infection include prolonged surgical time, postoperative hemorrhage, previous joint replacement, steroid use, and concurrent infection at the time of surgery, rheumatoid arthritis, obesity, and diabetes mellitus.

Most infections are caused by coagulase negative staphylococci and by *S. aureus* followed by Gram-negative bacilli, streptococci, enterococci, and fungi. There are three categories of prosthetic joint infections (Table 11.5). Management requires removal of hardware and the institution of intravenous antibiotics. A two-stage surgical replacement is the preferred approach because it has the highest success rate in terms of cure and functional outcome. For some pathogens and early-onset infections, many practitioners prefer either a one-stage approach combined with aggressive early intravenous antibiotic management followed by the use of suppressive antibiotics including rifampin, which has good biofilm penetration.

Acute and Chronic Osteomyelitis

Bone is highly resistant to infection. However, under certain circumstances it may become affected due to a large inoculum of bacteria, trauma/fracture, or due to foreign objects. Osteomyelitis is characterized by the progressive inflammatory destruction of bone and new apposition of bone. Acute osteomyelitis refers to an

TABLE 11.5 Categories of Prosthetic Joint Infections[a]

Categories	Core concepts
Early onset (within 3 months from surgery)	Fever, surgical site erythema, wound drainage, joint pain, and joint effusion. Joint infection can be confirmed by joint aspiration (usually>4200 cells/mm^3), positive Gram-stain and/or culture or through intraoperative tissue frozen section demonstrating inflammation of periprosthetic tissue. Most commonly caused by S. aureus and Gram-negative bacilli. Clinically significant cellulitis and the formation of a sinus tract with purulent discharge may develop in the course of the infection. Likely acquired during implantation of the prosthesis.
Delayed onset (3–24 months from surgery)	More likely to present with chronic pain without any other symptoms. Low-grade infection may cause implant loosening, persistent joint pain and it is usually caused by less virulent microorganisms (coagulase negative staphylococci and Propionibacterium. acnes)[b] Likely acquired during implantation of the prosthesis.
Late onset (more than 24 months from surgery)	More likely to present with chronic pain without any other symptoms. Acquired through secondary bacteremic seeding from a different source of bacteremia such as urinary tract infection, dental infection, cutaneous or respiratory infection

[a]Zimmerli W, Trampuz A, Ochsner PE. Prosthetic-joint infections. N Engl J Med 2004;**351**(16): 1645–1654
[b]There is a syndrome affecting prosthetic shoulder infection associated with Propionibacterium acnes whereby there is a characteristic hemorrhagic or erythematous discoloration of the surgical wound even in delayed cases.

infection when with less than 10 days from its onset. Clinical signs persisting for more than 10 days correlate roughly with chronic osteomyelitis and defined as the presence of necrotic bone. This distinction is important because the presence of necrotic bone requires its removal to promote healing and prevent further spread of the infectious process. The purulent process resulting from bacterial induced intraosseous inflammation spreads into vascular channels raising intraosseous pressure and impairing blood flow resulting in ischemic necrosis of bone with development of separation of devascularized fragments (sequestra). Neutrophilic infiltration, bacterial and congested and/or thrombosed blood vessels are considered the hallmarks of the pathologic findings in acute osteomyelitis. Chronic osteomyelitis is defined by the presence of necrotic bone with the absence of living osteocytes. Most common cause of osteomyelitis is S. aureus followed by coagulase negative staphylococci, Gram-negative bacilli including Pseudomonas aeruginosa, and Streptococcus spp. (Table 11.6). Osteomyelitis

TABLE 11.6 Core Concepts of Acute, Chronic[a] and Vertebral Osteomyelitis[b]

Type	Description	Core concepts
Acute	Short duration (<10 days) Other consider <30 days • Hematogenous (in children located in metaphyseal area of long bones (tibia and femur) but also in adults associated with community-associated USA300 Methicillin Resistant *S. aureus* (MRSA).[c] In hematogenous osteomyelitis surgery is usually not required • Contiguous (open fracture, or associated with joint prostheses) • Vascular insufficiency (diabetes mellitus)	*S. aureus* binds to fibronectin, laminin, collagen, and bone sialoglycoprotein through fibronectin binding adhesins *S. aureus* (most common cause in acute and chronic) Coagulase negative staphylococci (foreign body associated) Streptococci (diabetes mellitus, bites, decubitus ulcers) *Salmonella* (sickle cell disease) Bartonellosis (HIV) *Eikenella corrodens* (human bites) *Pasteurella* (dog/cat bites)
Chronic	Necrotic bone that requires debridement to promote healing • Contiguous (open fracture, or associated with joint prostheses) • Vascular insufficiency (diabetes mellitus)	Necrotic bone is the hallmark of chronic osteomyelitis. *S. aureus* can survive intracellularly in a metabolic altered state (small-colony variants) explaining its persistence in chronic infections and also explaining elevated failure rate with short courses of antibiotics
Vertebral (spinal osteomyelitis, spondylodiskitis, septic diskitis, or disk-space infection)	Acute • Hematogenous seeding[d] • Spinal surgery • Contiguous spread	*S. aureus and E. coli* coagulase negative staphylococci associated with infected pacemaker leads *P. acnes* and coagulase negative staphylococci *S. aureus*, coagulase negative staphylococci Gram-negative including *Pseudomonas* spp

TABLE 11.6 Core Concepts of Acute, Chronic and Vertebral Osteomyelitis (*cont.*)

Type	Description	Core concepts
	Chronic	Brucellosis Tuberculosis (Pott's disease) Q fever Pyogenic

[a]*Zimmerli W. Vertebral osteomyelitis. N Engl J Med 2010;362(11):1022–1029.*
[b]*Lew DP, Waldvogel FA. Osteomyelitis. N Engl J Med 1997;336(14):999–1007.*
[c]*Seybold U, Talati NJ, Kizilbash Q, Shah M, Blumberg HM, Franco-Paredes C. Hematogenous osteomyelitis mimicking osteosarcoma due to community-associated Methicillin-Resistant Staphylococcus aureus. Infection. 2007;35(3):190–193.*
[d]*Most patient with hematogenous vertebral osteomyelitis have underlying medical conditions including diabetes mellitus, coronary atherosclerotic heart disease, cancer, or are on hemodialysis. Also, patients may have a history of intravenous drug use (Gordon RJ, Lowy FD. Bacterial infections in drug users. N Engl J Med 2005;353(18):1945–1953).*

may develop through hematogenous seeding, due to a contiguous focus of infection, or due to vascular insufficiency.

Acute pyogenic vertebral osteomyelitis can be associated with infection of other contiguous compartments including epidural, paravertebral, and psoas abscesses. In as many as 25–50% of cases there is associated neurologic involvement with motor weakness or paralysis. Blood cultures are crucial in the diagnostic evaluation of vertebral osteomyelitis since 58–78% of cases have ongoing bacteremia. Alternatively, if blood cultures are not helpful in making a specific diagnosis, then CT scan imaging guided aspiration/biopsy for obtaining a specimen for Gram-staining and culture for bacterial, fungal, and mycobacterial pathogens prior to initiation of antibiotics, is therefore indicated. The reason *Escherichia coli* or sometimes-other Gram-negative organisms are identified in vertebral osteomyelitis is due to backflow of this pathogen in patients with urinary tract infections via Batson's venous plexus. This venous system is a valveless system that connects deep pelvic and thoracic veins to the internal vertebral venous plexuses (Table 11.6).

Complications of Chronic Osteomyelitis

Patients with chronic osteomyelitis may develop unusual complications as a result of the persistent inflammatory response associated with chronic infection. Secondary (reactive) amyloidosis may occur which may lead to renal amyloidosis with a secondary nephrotic syndrome (proteinuria, hypoalbuminemia, hypercoagulability, hyperlipidemia). Additionally, a verrucous cutaneous carcinoma may develop in the affected area surrounding a focus of chronic osteomyelitis.

DRUG-INDUCED BONE DISORDERS SEEN BY INFECTIOUS DISEASES CLINICIANS

Bisphosphonates and Osteonecrosis of the Jaw

The use of bisphosphonates has been associated with two conditions that often call for infectious diseases consultations. One of them is the occurrence a collapsing glomerulopathy, which sometimes has to be distinguished clinically and by laboratory with HIV-associated nephropathy (HIVAN), since this condition also produces a collapsing glomerulopathy.

Osteonecrosis of the jaw in patients with use of bisphosphonate therapy is a frequently seen condition by some infectious diseases clinicians.[2–4] Although its etiology is not caused by an infectious pathogen, it can complicate with secondary infection and its management often require the use of doxycycline and oral antiseptics. Management of this condition requires a multidisciplinary team including oral surgeons, oncologists, and infectious disease clinicians.[3]

The term bisphosphonate-related osteonecrosis of the jaw (BRONJ) comprises two categories: cancer and noncancer related. Bisphosphonates are drugs used in the treatment of multiple myeloma, hypercalcemia of malignancy, or sometimes used in the management of osteoporosis and Paget's disease.[3,4] The type, dose, and duration of bisphosphonate seem to play a role, with higher risk when these drugs are used intravenously and for prolonged periods of time. However, some patients may only have a brief exposure and developed a clinical picture of full-blown BRONJ. The postulated mechanism of damage occurs due to suppression of bone turnover and inability to repair bone micro damage (inhibition of the enzyme farnesyl diphosphate synthase in osteoclasts). In addition, the accumulation of these drugs may be sufficient to produce toxicity to the oral epithelium and to inhibit formation of new capillaries by inhibiting antiangiogenic properties. Local risk factors for triggering the onset of BRONJ include dentoalveolar surgery including dental extractions, dental implant placement, periapical surgery, and periodontal surgery involving osseous injury. Its localization to the jaw may have to do with the microbial environment in the oral cavity.[3]

Prevention of BRONJ is a priority and before starting therapy with bisphosphonates, ideally, patients should undergo a thorough oral examination. Treatment should include preservation of quality of life through control of pain, control of secondary infections, prevention of extension of lesion and development of new areas of necrosis. Patients with established BRONJ should avoid elective dentoalveolar surgical procedures. Most patients respond to long-term daily doxycycline and oral antimicrobial rinses with clorhexidine and meticulous home care oral hygiene. Secondary infection often requires prolonged courses of intravenous antibiotics.[2–4]

Tenofivir-Induced Osteopenia and Osteoporosis in HIV-Infected Individuals

Adding one more potential system involved in HIV-infection, low bone mineral density is common in HIV-infected individuals whether antiretroviral-treated or antiretroviral-naïve.[5] In addition, to the traditional risk factors for osteoporosis, HIV-infected individuals have alterations in bone metabolism not only due to antivirals, HIV-infection, but also due to chronic inflammation. Hepatitis C coinfection adds further risk to HIV in causing impairment of bone metabolism.

Tenofivir disoproxil fumarate (TDV),[5] the nucleotide reverse transcriptase inhibitor (NRTI) and the protease inhibitors are associated with greater bone losses than other antiretroviral drugs. Tenofivir can cause hypophosphatemia secondary to proximal renal tubular dysfunction triggering bone reabsorption and in some cases it may cause renal failure. Tenofivir alafenamide, a prodrug of tenofivir that it is metabolized intracellularly to TDV may decrease the risk of bone toxicity.[5]

REFERENCES

1. Zimmermann 3rd B, Mikolich DJ, Ho Jr G. Septic bursitis. *Semin Arthritis Rheum* 1995;**24**(6):391–410.
2. Vescovi P. Bisphosphonates and osteonecrosis: an open matter. *Clin Cases Miner Bone Metab* 2012;**9**(3):142–4.
3. Khan AA, Morrison A, Hanley DA, Felsenberg D, McCauley LK, O'Ryan F, et al. Diagnosis and management of osteonecrosis of the jaw: a systematic review and international consensus. *J Bone Miner Res* 2015;**30**(1):3–23.
4. Ruggiero SL, Dodson TB, Fantasia J, Goodday R, Aghaloo T, Mehrotra B, et al. American Association of Oral and Maxillofacial Surgeons position paper on medication-related osteonecrosis of the jaw-2014 update. *J Oral Maxillofac Surg* 2014;**72**(10):1938–56.
5. Hileman CO, Eckard AR, McComsey GA. Bone loss in HIV: a contemporary review. *Curr Opin Endocrinol Diabetes Obes* 2015;**22**(6):446–51.

Chapter 12

Nonsuppurative Manifestations of Infections

DIAGNOSTIC APPROACH TO NONSUPPURATIVE MANIFESTATIONS OF INFECTIOUS PATHOGENS

Rheumatic Fever

The classic nonsuppurative complications of *Streptococcus pyogenes* infection include acute rheumatic fever and glomerulonephritis. Other condition associated with *Streptococcus pyogenes* is the pediatric autoimmune neuropsychiatric disorders associated with streptococcal infections and linked to the spectrum of obsessive–compulsive disorders. Acute rheumatic fever is a nonsuppurative complication of pharyngeal infection with group A streptococci (GAS—*Streptococcus pyogenes*) eliciting a humoral and cell mediated immune responses to components of the bacterium which are immunologically similar to antigens (molecular mimicry) present in particular tissues (joints, heart, and central nervous system). The streptococcal M protein of some streptococcal strains has similar molecular properties as laminin and cardiac myosin and thus may be the triggering antigen in some cases. The clinical presentation of this disease appears characteristically 2–3 weeks after initial infection.[1] Most patients with rheumatic fever do not recall experiencing any sore throat the weeks preceding the onset of signs and symptoms consistent with rheumatic fever; and throat cultures are only positive for GAS in a minority of patients with acute rheumatic fever. Rheumatic fever in children predominantly manifests by involvement of the heart, whereas most adults manifest with abrupt onset of polyarthralgias and fever. Some patients have the classic migratory pattern but there are other conditions that may produce a migratory pattern (see chapter: Osteoarticular Infections). In addition, rheumatic nodules and erythema marginatum are rarely seen in adults since they tend to be linked to the occurrence of carditis (Table 12.1). Current estimates of the global burden of acute rheumatic fever and rheumatic heart disease continue to demonstrate a substantial impact but the precise estimates are difficult to establish.[2] Most cases occur in Asia, Australia, and the Middle East.[2] Laboratory diagnosis of rheumatic fever can be also confirmed with positive antibody

Core Concepts in Clinical Infectious Diseases (CCCID). http://dx.doi.org/10.1016/B978-0-12-804423-0.00012-3

TABLE 12.1 Rheumatic Fever Clinical Criteria (Jones Criteria)[a]

Major manifestations	Minor manifestations	Supporting evidence of streptococcal Infection
Carditis	Previous rheumatic fever or	Positive oropharyngeal
Polyarthritis	rheumatic heart disease	culture for *S. pyogenes*
Chorea	Arthralgias	Titers of antistreptolysin
Erythema marginatum	Fever	consistent with *S. pyo-*
Subcutaneous nodules	*Laboratory:*	*genes* infection
		Recent episode of scarlet
	Elevated erythrocyte	fever
	sedimentations rate (ESR)	
	Elevated C-reactive protein	
	Prolonged P–R interval in	
	the electrocardiogram	
	Leukocytosis	

[a]*The presence of two major criteria, or of one major and two minor criteria, is highly suggestive of rheumatic fever, if supported by evidence of preceding group A streptococcal infection (Dajani AS. Current status of non-suppurative complications of groups A streptococci. Pediatr Infect Dis J 1991;**10**(10):S25–S27).*

response to antistreptolysin. However, antibody titers may not indicate recent infection since they can remain elevated for many months.

Reactive Syndromes

Acute rheumatic fever and poststreptococcal reactive arthritis have different clinical manifestations (Table 12.2). In some individuals, after an episode of enteritis/gastroenteritis/enterocolitis caused by either *Salmonella, Shigella, Campylobacter*, or *Yersinia* may result in an asymmetric additive polyarthritis involving predominantly the large joints in lower extremities. Similarly urogenital infection (sexually acquired) caused mainly by *Chlamydia trachomatis* may lead to the same manifestations. A minority of patients with arthritis associated with genital infections have the triad of conjunctivitis, urethritis, and arthritis (previously Reiter's syndrome) (see chapter: Osteoarticular Infections). Symptoms may begin with entesophathy (pain tendon insertion site), dactylitis (sausage digits) followed by large joint affection and most commonly occurring 1 or 2 weeks after the initial enterocolitic or urogenital clinical presentation. Some patients may experience postviral reactive arthritis. The most relevant viral pathogen that induced a long-term postinfectious syndrome is chikungunya with severe arthralgias in many patients; and often synovitis in a minority of cases. Other alpha-viruses (togaviruses) may produce a postinfectious arthritis/arthralgia syndrome. Infection caused by *Mycobacterium tuberculosis* may be related to a spectrum of inflammatory (reactive) syndromes (Table 12.3).

TABLE 12.2 Differences between Rheumatic Fever and Poststreptococcal Reactive Arthritis[a]

Acute rheumatic fever	Poststreptococcal reactive arthritis
Patients are of young age	Patients are of older age
Longer interval between group A streptococci infection an onset of clinical manifestations (2–3 weeks)	Shorter interval between group A streptococci infection an onset of arthritis (<10 days)
Patients require monthly injections with benzyl penicillin for at least 5 years after the diagnosis of acute rheumatic fever and in the presence of cardiac valvular abnormalities, secondary prophylaxis should be used for prolonged periods	Patients respond much less to salicylates
	Arthritis is additive, nonmigratory and frequently chronic (>6 weeks in more than 50% of patients)
	Elevation of inflammatory markers (C-reactive protein and erythrocyte sedimentation rate)
Arthritis affects large joints and sometimes migratory (sometimes Jaccoud's arthropathy) but is self-limiting	Arthritis affects large joints
Fever is often present	Fever is often present
Elevation of inflammatory markers (C-reactive protein and erythrocyte sedimentation rate)	Both genders may be equally affected
Females are more frequently affected	Erythema nodosum
Erythema marginatum	Cardiac involvement has been described in children
Carditis and valvular heart disease are often present. Carditis is present in the youngest children and decreasing with increasing age	No increased risk of valvular heart disease in adults
Valvular heart disease peaks at 25–34 years as a result of acute rheumatic fever during childhood	No evidence of increased morbidity, however, significant morbidity associated with chronic arthritis
Increased mortality due to valvular heart disease	Can also be caused by group C or G streptococci
Only caused by group A streptococci	

[a]Clinical and laboratory distinction is important since treatment and prognosis is different. Indeed, both conditions represent two different clinical entities with different clinical outcomes (Van der Helm-van Mil AHM. Acute rheumatic fever and poststreptococcal reactive arthritis reconsidered. Curr Opin Rheumatol 2010;**22**:437–442).

GLOMERULONEPHRITIS

The epidemiology of glomerulonephritis associated with bacterial pathogens is transitioning from being mostly associated with streptococci to now resulting more frequently from staphylococci and Gram-negative bacilli. However, different infectious agents can be associated with glomerulonephritis (GN)[3,4] (Table 12.4). Some strains of group A streptococci can

TABLE 12.3 Tuberculosis Related Inflammatory Diseases[a]

Category[b]	Description
Reactive immunologic phenomena	Poncet's reactive arthritis Erythema nodosum Erythema induratum (Bazin's erythema) Amyloidosis (AA type) Uveitis
Drug-induced syndromes	Fluoroquinolone induced tendinopathy Uveitis induced by rifamycins Drug-induced lupus by isoniazid or rifamycins Hyperuricemia/Gout induced by pyrazinamide

[a]Franco-Paredes C, Diaz-Borjon A, Barragán L, Senger M, Leonard M. The ever-expanding association between tuberculosis and rheumatologic diseases. Am J Med 2006;**119**:470–477.
[b]Additionally, tuberculosis may cause other inflammatory but septic conditions such as septic arthritis, spondylitis, myositis, subcutaneous abscess, tenosynovitis; and through the use of immunosuppressive agents in the treatment of rheumatoid arthritis patients may developed active tuberculosis.

TABLE 12.4 Infections Associated with Glomerulonephritis

Type	Type of glomerulonephritis	Core concepts
Viral		
HIV	HIVAN (collapsing FSGS and microcystic changes in renal tubules)[a]	Affects mostly African-American individuals (genetic marker APOL1 in chromosome 22) and HIVAN is the most common cause of chronic kidney disease in HIV-infected individuals. Antiretroviral therapy is beneficial to slow progression[b,c]
Hepatitis C	Type I Membranoproliferative in hepatitis C	
Hepatitis B	Membranous Nephropathy in hepatitis B	Rarely, membranoproliferative GN
Enterovirus (ECHO and Coxackie B)	FSGS	
Herpes viruses (cytomegalovirus, Varicella–Zoster virus, Epstein–Barr virus) Mumps Rubella	FSGS	

TABLE 12.4 Infections Associated with Glomerulonephritis (*cont.*)

Type	Type of glomerulonephritis	Core concepts
Influenza Parvovirus B 19[c], Simian virus 40	FSGS	
Parasitic (helminths)		
Filarial (*Wuchereria bancrofti, Brugia malayi, Loa loa, Onchocerca volvulus*)	Diffuse GN and membranoproliferative GN, minimal change and chronic sclerosing GN	Patients with parasite-related GN be treated with effective antiparasitic therapy and avoid use of steroids or immunosuppressive drugs. Effective treatment improves renal disease outcomes
Trematodes (*Schistosoma mansoni, S. haematobium, S. japonicum*)	Classification: 1. Mesangial profileration/ focal proliferative/diffuse proliferative 2. Exudative 3. Mesangiocapillary type I 4. FSGS 5. Amyloidosis	Schistosomal nepropahty should be treated with praziquantel and avoid steroid use. Blood cultures for *Salmonella* are indicated since coinfection worsens renal disease and treatment of typhoidal or nontyphoidal *Salmonella* spp improves clinical outcomes of schistosoma-induced renal disease
Protozoal (*Plasmodium malariae, Plasmodium falciparum, Leishmania donovani, Toxoplasma gondii, Trypanosoma cruzi, Trypanosoma brucei rhodesiense*)	*P. malariae* (and to a lesser extent *P. vivax* and *P. ovale*) are associated with membranous nephropathy and membranoproliferative GN, while *P. falciparum* may cause acute kidney injury or proliferative GN	Antimalarial treatment improves clinical outcomes. Avoid steroids and immunosuppressive drugs

(Continued)

TABLE 12.4 Infections Associated with Glomerulonephritis (*cont.*)

Type	Type of glomerulonephritis	Core concepts
Bacterial		
Streptococci (*S. pneumoniae*, viridans-group-streptococci, *S. pyogenes*)	Endocapillary GN with mesangial and capillary granular immune deposition	Acute nephritic syndrome usually lasts 2 weeks. In a minority of children, disease may progress to crescentic disease with rapidly progressive kidney dysfunction. Persistent hypocomplementemia after 3 months require kidney biopsy to rule out membranoproliferative GN
Mycobacterial (*Mycobacterium leprae, M. tuberculosis*)	Chronic infection due to *M. leprae* or *M. tuberculosis* may develop amyloidosis (AA)	
Salmonella (*S.* Typhi, *S.* Paratyphi, *S.* Typhimurium) Treponemal (Syphilis) *Yersinia enterocolitica Brucella abortus Coxiella burnetti Listeria monocytogenes Corynebacterium diphteriae Leptospira interrogans*	Diffuse GN and membrano-proliferative GN, minimal change and chronic scle-rosing GN	
Staphylococcus aureus and coagulase negative staphylococci	*Staphylococcus aureus* is currently more frequently associated with GN than with viridans group streptococci. Focal segmental proliferative GN often associated with focal crescents is characteristic of patients with infective endocarditis. However, some patients may present with diffuse proliferative endocapillary lesion with our without crescents	Most likely occurring during an episode of infective endocarditis. Prognosis is excellent with treatment of endocarditis and usually improving after 4–6 weeks of intravenous antibiotics. *Staphylococci* are also associated with shunt nephritis

TABLE 12.4 Infections Associated with Glomerulonephritis (*cont.*)

Type	Type of glomerulonephritis	Core concepts
Fungi (*Histoplasma capsulatum, Candida* spp, *Coccidiodes immitis*)	Membranous and membranoproliferative GN	

GN, Glomerulonephritis; FSGS, focal segmental glomerular sclerosis.

[a]*The spectrum of kidney disease in HIV-infected individuals is broad: HIVAN-collapsing FSGS, aterionephrosclerosis, immune complex GN (membranoproliferative pattern of injury or lupus like GN), idiopathic FSGS, HCV and cryoglobulinemia, thrombotic microangiopathies, membranous nephropathy (HBV) or malignancy associated, IgA nephropathy, diabetic nephropathy, postinfectious (infective endocarditis or other infectious processes), crystal nephropathy (protease inhibitors, acyclovir, sulfadiazine), proximal tubulopathy-Fanconi like syndrome (tenofivir disoproxil fumarate), acute tubular necrosis.*

[b]*Virus associated (may affect the podocyte directly or through cytokine release by inflammatory cytokines). HIV (HIVAN) is produced by direct infection of podocytes and tubular epithelial cells by HIV. HIV-1 produced proteins nef and vpr dysregulates renal epithelium leading to FSG and rapidly progressing to glomerular collapse (a similar phenomenon occurs due to bisphosphonate therapy).*

[c]*HIV-1 can persist in the kidney epithelium despite the institution of antiretroviral therapy and measured virologic suppression and immune recovery. HIV-synthetized proteins in tubular cells lead to glomular collapse. HIV-protein nef is major virulence factors that promotes podocyte dedifferentiation and proliferation and dysregulation of actin cytoskeleton of podocytes. Whereas, the vpr protein mediates tubular epithelial G2 cell arrest and apoptosis. All this pathogenic mechanisms result in glomerular collapse manifesting as severe kidney injury. Parvovirus B19 can infect podocytes and tubular cells leading to FSG.*

produce acute glomerulonephritis and this risk is associated with some strains bearing certain M proteins (nephritogenic such as M protein type 49). Acute glomerulonephritis (crescentic) typically occurs 4–6 weeks after streptococci pyoderma or 7–14 days after an episode of pharyngitis. However, cutaneous pyodermas are the main streptococci syndrome associated with acute glomerulonephritis. In addition to group A streptococci, group C streptococci (*Streptococcus dysgalactiae subspecies equisimilis* or *Streptococcus anginosus*) may be associated with glomerulonephritis. However, infection due to group C or group G streptococci (*Streptococcus dysgalactiae subspecies equisimilis* or *Streptococcus anginosus*) are not associated with rheumatic fever. The disease is precipitated by antigen–antibody complexes deposition on the glomerular basement membrane. Soluble streptococcal antigens are considered the inciting agent. Reinfection with streptococci may rarely leads to a recurrence of acute glomerulonephritis. Patients may present with a nephritic syndrome picture and evidence of hypocomplementemia (decreased levels of C3). Short-term prognosis of the acute phase of post-streptococcal GN is excellent in the majority of children, but in the elderly mortality may be as high as 20%. Management requires penicillin or erythromycin. Regarding the nephritic syndrome, diuretics and antihypertensive drugs are sometimes required. Pulses of intravenous methylprednisolone should be considered in patients with rapidly progressive crescentic GN.

GLOMERULONEPHRITIS ASSOCIATED WITH INFECTIVE BACTERIAL ENDOCARDITIS

Relevant risk factors for the development of GN associated with infective endocarditis include intravenous drug use, prosthetic heart valves, and structural heart disease[3,4] (Table 12.4). *Staphylococcus aureus* is currently more frequently associated with GN than with viridans group streptococci. Focal segmental proliferative GN often associated with focal crescents is characteristic of patients with infective endocarditis. However, some patients may present with diffuse proliferative endocapillary lesion with our without crescents.

MEMBRANOPROLIFERATIVE GN ASSOCIATED WITH VENTRICULAR SHUNTS

This condition results from an immune complex-mediated GN that develops as a complication of chronic infection of ventriculoatrial, or ventriculojugular shunts inserted for the management of hydrocephalus. Patients developed a nephritic syndrome (hypertension, azotemia, proteinuria, and hematuria) with prolonged fever. Histologically it typically presents with a type-1 membranoproliferative GN with granular deposits of IgM, IgG, C3, and electron-dense mesangial and subendothelial deposits. Infection is present in more than 30% of shunts and usually with staphylococci. Ventriculoperitoneal shunts are rarely complicated with shunt nephritis. Prognosis is excellent with early diagnosis, antibiotic therapy, and shunt removal.

VIRAL-INDUCED FOCAL SEGMENTAL GLOMERULOSCLEROSIS

A nephrotic syndrome picture accompanies focal segmental glomerulosclerosis (FSG) and characterized as proteinuria, peripheral edema, hypoalbuminemia, and hyperlipidemia (hypercholesterolemia). The cardinal feature of FSG is glomerular scarring that begins with focal sclerosis (involving a minority of glomeruli) and segmental (affection a portion of the glomerular globe). Eventually, more global and widespread glomerulosclerosis ensues. The podocytes are the cellular target of injury and disease in FSG. There are primary and secondary forms of FSG. Of the secondary forms, familial or genetic are associated with mutation in specific podocyte proteins. Other secondary forms include: drug induced (heroin, interferons, bisphosphonates, anabolic steroids, or calcineurin-inhibitor); adaptive to elevated body–mass index, systemic hypertension, and other conditions; and virus associated (Table 12.4). Thrombotic events complicate the nephrotic syndrome in approximately 25% of cases due to urinary loss anticoagulation proteins (antithrombin II) and increased synthesis of procoagulant factors leading to a hypercoagulable state.[5]

MEMBRANOPROLIFERATIVE GLOMERULONEPHRITIS ASSOCIATED WITH HEPATITIS C VIRUS

Kidney involvement in hepatitis C infection (HCV) is usually associated with type II cryoglobulinemia and manifests clinically as a nephritic syndrome with moderate kidney insufficiency.[3,4] Histologically there is a characteristic type I membranoproliferative GN with deposition of IgM, IgG, C3 in the mesangium and capillary walls on immunofluorescence. In addition, a vasculitis of the small- and medium-size renal arteries may be present. Other glomerular disease that can be associated with HCV includes: thrombotic microangiopathies, focal segmental glomerulosclerosis, IgA nephropathy, fibrillary and immunotactoid GN, membranous nephropathy. Sustained virologic response with new therapies improves clinical outcomes of glomerulopathies associated with hepatitis C (Table 12.4).

MEMBRANOUS NEPHROPATHY ASSOCIATED WITH HEPATITIS B VIRUS

Hepatitis B virus infection (HBV) may be associated with membranous nephropathy, membranoproliferative GN, FSGS, and IgA nephropathy.[4] The most commonly identified form histopathologically is membranous nephropathy, particularly in children. In adults, HBV-mediated GN is a progressive disease and patients usually present with nephrotic syndrome. Treatment of hepatitis B with nucleoside or nucleotide analogs is indicated to improve clinical outcomes of renal involvement by HBV (Table 12.4).

AMYLOIDOSIS

Amyloidosis (AA type) may complicate chronic infections processes or chronic inflammatory diseases such as rheumatoid arthritis. Chronic infectious diseases classically associated with AA amyloidosis include tuberculosis, leprosy, and brucellosis given the long-term inflammation associated with *M. tuberculosis* and *M. leprae*, respectively. Chronic parasitic infections can also lead to renal amyloidosis such as *Schistosoma mansoni* or *Schistosoma haematobium*.[5] It usually manifests as an organ-specific amyloidosis, such as nephritic or nephrotic syndrome, cardiac amyloidosis, hepatic amyloidosis, or nerve infiltration. Chronic osteomyelitis and bronchiectasis can also be associated with renal amyloidosis. HIV infection has also been associated with amyloidosis cardiac amyloidosis.[6,7]

TOXIN-MEDIATED DISEASES

This group of conditions arise usually by ingestion of bacteria with production of toxin in the intestinal tract or ingestion of the toxin (intoxication) (Table 12.5).

TABLE 12.5 Toxin-Mediated Manifestations of Infectious Diseases

Staphylococcus aureus	Toxic shock syndrome Bullous impetigo Scalded skin syndrome (Ritter's disease) Food Poisoning	TSST-1 (Superantigens) Exfoliative exotoxin (epidermolytic) Exfoliative exotoxin (epidermolytic toxin A and B) Enterotoxins
Streptococcus pyogenes	Toxic shock syndrome Scarlet fever[a] Pharyngitis tonsillitis	Pyrogenic exotoxin A Consists of usually pharyngitis accompanied by a papular rash (minute – sand paper like) due to pyrogenic exotoxins A, B, and C (erythrogenic or scarlet fever toxins). Associated findings circumoral pallor, strawberry tongue, and accentuation of the rash in skin folds (Pastia's lines)
Archanobacterium haemolyticum	Pharyngitis tonsillitis (toxin not defined)	Maculopapular rash blanching (scarlatiniform). Scarlet fever is more papular
Clostridium botulinum	Botulism (BoNT/A and B)	Descending paralysis with involvement of cranial nerves
Clostridium tetani	Tetanus (TeNT)	Hyperexcitability and Autonomic dysfunction
Clostridium histiotoxic syndromes (more than 10 toxins that are associated with a spectrum of disease that range from localized wound contamination to overwhelming systemic disease	*C. perfringens* (alpha-toxin, perfringolysin) *C. septicum* (alpha-toxin –lecithinase) *C. histolyticum* (collagenases) *C. novy* (alpha-novyi) *C. haemolyticum* (beta-hemolysin) *C. sordellii* (TcsL, TcsH)	Disease is mediated by toxins and includes soft tissue infections such as gas gangrene (*C. perfringens*), enteric diseases such as food poisoning, enteritis necroticans, antibiotic associated colitis (*C. difficile*), and neutropenic enterocolitis (*C. septicum*) and neurologic syndromes (tetanus and botulism). *C. septicum* can cause spontaneous nontraumatic gas gangrene, *C. sordelii* gas gangrene of the uterus, bacteremias (*C. perfringens*) and polymicrobial severe infections
Bacillus cereus	Food poisoning (emetic toxin and three enterotoxins)	Rapid onset after ingestion of contaminated rice of nausea, vomiting and diarrhea

TABLE 12.5 Toxin-Mediated Manifestations of Infectious Diseases (*cont.*)

Mycobacterium ulcerans	Mycolactone	Buruli ulcer causing subcutaneous and fatty tissue necrosis
Shigella dysenteriae and Escherichia coli	Shiga-toxin hemolytic uremic syndrome (ST-HUS)	Thrombotic Microangiopathy (hemolytic uremic syndrome) most commonly seen in children typically with acute kidney injury, most cases are sporadic but large outbreaks also may occur
Intoxications mimicking infectious diseases	Scombroid food poisoning (histidine converted to histamine)	Acquired from ingestion of spoiled fish (mimicks allergy) since histidine is converted to histamine in decaying fish (mackerel, bonito, tuna)
	Ciguatera food poisoning (ciguatoxin) Systemic marine toxins	Ciguatoxin produced by benthic dinoflagellates (*Gambierdiscus*) growing in association with microalgae in reefs and subsequently ingested by fish, which in turn is ingested by humans (reef fish: barracuda, mahi mahi) and produces circumoral paresthesias, nausea, vomiting, diarrhea, and neurologic and neuropsychiatric symptoms
	Pfeisteria pisciscida (possible estuary-associated syndrome)	Possible exposure through aerosolized toxin or skin causing cognitive and visual changes that improve with cholestyramine. This may occur in Atlantic coast in the United States
Entertoxigenic *Escherichia coli*	Watery diarrhea (traveler's diarrhea)	Toxin induces active secretion
Vibrio cholerae 01	Cholera toxin (subunit A/B)	Cholera with severe dehydration and volume depletion in endemic areas and during pandemics
Diphteria	Corynebacterium diphteriae	Toxin induces protein synthesis leading to myocarditis, neuritis, and other life-threatening complications

[a]*Differential diagnosis of Scarlet fever include Kawasaki's disease, toxic shock syndrome, drug-reaction, measles, and other viral exanthems.*

MALIGNANCIES ASSOCIATED WITH INFECTIOUS DISEASES

There is an important association between some infectious pathogens and neo-plastic disorders.[8] This may as a result of reduced surveillance immunopro-tective mechanisms among immunocompromised individuals. However, there are also some microorganisms that elicit a chronic inflammatory response that subsequently results in malignant transformation. In addition, other organisms are directly oncogenic such as some viral pathogens (Table 12.6).

TABLE 12.6 Malignancies Associated with Infectious Diseases

Category	Associated malignancies	Key issues
Carcinomas	HIV (head and neck, lung, breast, ovarian) EBV (nasopharyngeal, head and neck) Hepatitis B (chronic hepatitis B or cirrhosis associated hepatocarcinoma) Hepatitis C (cirrhosis associated hepatocarcinoma) Nontyphoidal *Salmonella* (ie, *S.* Typhimurium) (gallbladder carcinoma) *Schistosoma haematobium* (squamous cell carcinoma of the bladder) Osteomyelitis (Marjorlin's ulcer (verrucous squamous cell cutaneous carcinoma which may occur with long-lasting pressure ulcers, stasis ulcers, burn scars) Human papillomavirus (HPV) (cervical, penile, oropharyngeal, and rectal carcinomas)	Although there are some malignancies classically associated with HIV-infection (eg, Kaposi's sarcoma) given the fact that patients are living longer and may have risk factors for other non-HIV related malignancies, there is an increasing incidence of many carcinomas (eg, lung, anal, and others)[a] Polyomavirus such as Merkel cell polyomavirus (MCPyV) has been linked to Merkel cell carcinoma, which is a neuroendocrine carcinoma
Adenocarcinoma	*H. pylori* (stomach) and esophagus (due to overtreating *H. pylori*)[b]	
Sarcomas (smooth muscle tumors)[a]	Epstein–Barr virus (EBV) and HIV coinfection	Leiomyoma Leiomyosarcoma (mostly in children with HIV/ EBV co-infection[c]
Lymphomas	Epstein–Barr virus (Burkitt's lym-phoma and posttransplantation lymphoproliferative disorder) Hepatitis C (splenic lymphoma as-sociated with cryoglobulinemia)	

TABLE 12.6 Malignancies Associated with Infectious Diseases (*cont.*)

Category	Associated malignancies	Key issues
	Human herpes virus 8 (HHV-8) (body-cavity lymphoma) coinfection with HIV	HHV-8 can also be associated with multicentric Castleman's disease which is characterized by plasmacytic lymphadenopathy with polyclonal hyperglobulinemia and elevated levels of interleukin-6 but it is not considered a malignancy
Leukemia	HTLV-1 (adult T-cell leukemia and lymphoma)	There are different forms: acute lymphomatous, chronic, and smouldering and more recently a primary cutaneous tumoral form.[d] Most patients present lymphadenopathy, hypercalcemia, hepatosplenomegaly; and multiple organ involvement (lungs, gastrointestinal tract and central nervous system)
MALTomas (mucosa-associated lymphoid tissue) considered a form of lymphoma originating from B cells in the marginal zone of the MALT	*H. pylori*, Hepatitis C	Treatment of *H. pylori* or hepatitis C improves clinical outcomes of MALTomas In some individuals, Helicobacter pylori may induce ulcerations of the gastric or duodenal mucosa unrelated to malignancies but that may lead to perforation peritonitis or gastrointestinal hemorrhage

[a]Brickman C, Palefsky JM. Cancer in the HIV-Infected host: epidemiology and pathogenesis in the antiretroviral era. Curr HIV/AIDS Rep 2015;PMID:26475669.
[b]Blaser M. Stop the killing of beneficial bacteria. Nature 2011;**476**:393–394.
[c]Purgina B, Rao UNM, Miettinen M, Pantanowitz L. AIDS-related EBV-associated smooth muscle tumors: a review of 64 published cases. Pathol Res Intern 2011;561548:1–10.
[d]Verdonck K, Gonzalez E, Van Dooren S, Vandamme AM, Vanham G, Gotuzzo E. Human T-lymphotropic virus 1: recent knowledge about an ancient infection. Lancet Infect Dis 2007;**7**:266–281.

TABLE 12.7 Established Causes of Systemic Vasculitis Associated with Infectious Diseases[a]

Size of blood vessel	Type of vasculitis	Associated infectious disease
Large vessel vasculitis	Giant cell arteritis (temporal arteritis) Takayasu's arteritis[b]	Varicella–Zoster virus[c] Some association with tuberculosis in Japan
Medium-size arteries	Polyarteritis nodosa	Association with hepatitis B. It has also been associated with hepatitis C, and hairy cell leukemia
Small vessel vasculitis	Type II cryoglobulinemia Henoch–Schönlein purpura	Hepatitis C *Streptococcus pyogenes pharyngitis Staphylococcus aureus bacteremia Helicobacter pylori* HIV Varicella–Zoster virus

[a]*Multiple bacterial pathogens including* Salmonella, Treponema pallidum *(syphilis) and rickettsia that are associated with inflammatory vasculopathies. In this context, we are referring to established systemic vasculitis and their associations with specific infectious pathogens. Many of these pathogens produce damage to the vessel wall by causing inflammation of the vaso vasorum and some may even cause mycotic aneurysms.*
[b]*Aggarwal A, Chag M, Sinha M, Naik S. Takayasu's arteritis: role of Mycobacterium tuberculosis and its 65 kDa heat shock protein. Int J Cardiol 1996;55(1):49–55.*
[c]*Powel DR 2nd, Patel S, Franco-Paredes C. Varicella-Zoser virus vasculopathy: the growing association between herpes zoster and strokes. Am J Med Sci 2015;350(3):243–245.*

SYSTEMIC VASCULITIS

Vasculitis is the inflammation of blood vessel walls that can lead to narrowing, ischemia, or development of aneurysms. Inflammation can affect small, medium, or large vessels and thus the classification of vasculitis is based on the size of the vessel (Table 12.7).

REFERENCES

1. Casey JD, Solomon DH, Gaziano TA, Miller AL, Loscalzo J. A patient with migrating polyarthralgias. *N Engl. J Med* 2013;**369**(1):75–80.
2. De Dassel JL, Ralph AP, Carapetis JR. Controlling acute rheumatic fever and rheumatic heart disease in developing countries: are we getting closer? *Curr Opin Pediatr* 2015;**27**:116–23.
3. D'Agati VD, Kaskel FJ, Falk RJ. Focal segmental glomerulosclerosis. *N Engl J Med* 2011;**363**(25):2398–411.

4. Kidney Inter Suppl (2011). Chapter 9. Infection-related glomerulonephritis. *Kidney Inter Suppl* 2012;**2**:200–8.
5. Loscalzo J. Venous thrombosis in the nephrotic syndrome. *N Engl J Med* 2013;**368**(10):956–7.
6. Amarawardena WKMG, Wijesundere A, Manohari HAD. Amyloidosis associated with HIV Infection. *Ceylon Med J* 2013;**58**:128–9.
7. Abdallah E, Waked E. Incidence and clinical outcome of renal amyloidosis: a retrospective study. *Saudi J Kidney Dis Transpl* 2013;**24**(5):950–8.
8. Ewald PW, Swain Ewald HA. Infection and cancer in multicellular organisms. *Phil Trans R Soc* 2015;**370**:20140224.

Chapter 13

Inflammatory and Autoimmune Syndromes Mimickers of Infection

DIAGNOSTIC APPROACH TO INFLAMMATORY AND AUTOIMMUNE CONDITIONS MIMICKING AN INFECTIOUS DISEASE

For the most part, autoimmunity and autoinflammation are the two mechanisms that may potentially present a challenge to clinicians in distinguishing infectious diseases from noninfectious inflammatory conditions. It is not a coincidence that there is an overlap in clinical manifestations between infectious diseases and inflammatory diseases. Indeed, signs and symptoms such as fever, cough, weight loss, generalized malaise, decreased appetite, elevated inflammatory serum markers, and other signs and symptoms may occur due to the activation of the innate and/or the acquired adaptive immune paths by either an infectious pathogen or a noninfectious inflammatory stimuli (and sometimes microorganisms).

AUTOIMMUNITY

Autoimmunity is characterized by self-directed inflammation, whereby aberrant dendritic cell, B and T-cell lymphocytes, responses in primary and secondary lymphoid organs lead to breaking of tolerance, with development of immune reactivity towards native antigens. In this instance, the innate immune response plays the predominant role in the clinical expression of the disease.[1] Systemic lupus erythemathosus (SLE) is the prototypic example of an autoimmune disease.

AUTOINFLAMMATION

Different from autoimmunity, autoinflammation is the self-directed inflammatory processes, whereby local factors at sites predisposed to disease leading to activation of innate immune cells, including macrophages and neutrophils with resultant tissue damage. Tissue microdamage predisposes an individual to site-specific inflammation that is independent of adaptive immune responses.

Core Concepts in Clinical Infectious Diseases (CCCID). http://dx.doi.org/10.1016/B978-0-12-804423-0.00013-5

157

For example, disturbed homeostasis of the cytokine cascade as it occurs in the periodic fevers syndromes (eg, familial Mediterranean fever).[2]

Clinicians often have to make a distinction between infectious and noninfectious causes of specific clinical syndromes such as it occurs in those with persistent and unexplained causes of fever, a condition that we define as fever of unknown origin or undifferentiated fever[3–8] (also see chapter: Febrile Syndromes). However, there are other important syndromes that fall into the category of non-infectious inflammatory pathologies that may potentially imitate many of the clinical manifestations of a well-defined infectious disease (Table 13.1).[3–8] Some of the categories of noninfectious inflammatory syndromes include: (1) neutrophilic dermatoses (Table 13.2); (2) eosinophilic skin diseases (Table 13.3); (3) pulmonary and eosinophilia syndromes (Table 13.4); and (4) neutrophilic dermatoses (Table 13.5).

TABLE 13.1 Common Noninfectious Inflammatory Syndromes that May Mimic Infectious Diseases[a]

Category	Description	Core concepts
Drug fever/ hyperthermia	Neuroleptic malignant syndrome	Associated with dopamine blockers (antipsychotic medications)
	Serotoninergic syndrome	Associated with selective serotoninergic reuptake inhibitors (SSRI) and monoamine oxidase inhibitors (linezolid)
	Common drugs inducing isolated fever	Phenytoin, sulfa drugs (trimethoprim-sulfamethoxazole, colace)
	Drug reaction eosinophilic systemic syndrome	Often due to allopurinol, penicillin, cephalosporins. Life-threatening reaction often causing acute kidney injury, transaminitis, hyperbilirubinemia and fever (differential diagnosis in this case include leptospirosis, and acute liver failure)
Thrombotic microangiopathies	*Escherichia coli/ Shigella dysenteriae*-associated thrombotic microangiopathies (ST-HUS)	Hemolytic uremic syndrome (mostly in children)
	ADAMTS13-associated thrombotic microangiopahty	Most commonly associated with HIV/AIDS. May also be triggered by drugs (quinine, cyclosporine, ticlopidine, clopidrogel, valacyclovir)

TABLE 13.1 Common Noninfectious Inflammatory Syndromes that May Mimic Infectious Diseases[a] (cont.)

Category	Description	Core concepts
Eosinophil activation syndromes	Pulmonary eosinophilia syndromes	Eosinophilic pneumonias Tropical pulmonary eosinophilia Drug-induced eosinophilia with pulmonary infiltrates (eg, nitrofurantoin)
	Eosinophilic skin diseases	Urticarial vasculitis, dermatitis herpetiformis, allergic drug eruption, eosinophilic granulomatosis with polyangiitis (Churg–Strauss), IgG-4 related disease, Wells syndrome, Gleich's syndrome, bullous pemphigoid, or Kimura's disease
Systemic vasculitis	Giant cell arteritis (GCA) Aortic arch vasculitis Takayasu's Polymyalgia rheumatica Drug-induced hypersensitivity vasculitis (beta-lactam antibiotics are frequent culprit) Henoch–Schönlein purpura (*Staphylococcus aureus* or *Streptococcus pyogenes* pharyngitis or viral infection induced) *ANCA-associated vasculitis:* Polyarteritis nodosa Granulomatosis and polyangiitis Microscopic polyangitis Churg–Strauss syndrome	Some diagnostic clues include presence of bruits, anemia of chronic inflammation, unexplained and recurrent episodes of fever without identifying a specific reason. Most frequent cause of fever of unknown origin in adults is temporal arteritis (GCA) manifested as fever, weight loss, decreased appetite, jaw claudication, decreased vision, temporal artery tenderness or skin lesion(s) in the territory of the temporal artery that could resemble trigeminal shingles. PMR usually presents in those younger than 50 years of age with shoulder and hip pain associated with episodic fever and anemia and chronic inflammation associated with elevated inflammatory markers[b]

(Continued)

TABLE 13.1 Common Noninfectious Inflammatory Syndromes that May Mimic Infectious Diseases[a] (cont.)

Category	Description	Core concepts
Macrophage activation syndromes	Systemic juvenile idiopathic arthritis (sJIA) Systemic lupus Erythematosus (SLE) Kawasaki's disease	Syndrome of fever, pancytopenia, hepatosplenomegaly, hypertriglyceridemia, transaminitis, and elevated ferritin levels (particularly in systemic juvenile idiopathic arthritis, the AOSD form in younger individuals, hemophagocytic syndrome, and in AOSD)
	Hemophagocytic Syndromes	Could be primary hemophagocytosis or infection-associated (most common causes include viral (Epstein-Barr virus, HIV) or fungal (disseminated histoplasmosis). Patients usually present with hyperferritinemia and elevated LDH
Cutaneous erythema syndromes	Erythema nodosum Erythema marginatum	Reactive to infection or medications Characteristic of rheumatic fever
	Erythema Induratum	Vasculitis nodular lesions associated with hypersensitivity to recent *Mycobacterium tuberculosis* infection
	Erythema elevatum diutinum	It is a form of leukocytoclastic vasculitis associated with IgA paraproteinemia and usually presenting in the knee and responds to dapsone
	Erythema multiforme	Well-defined targetoid (target-like) and annular lesions due to a drug reaction and sometimes due to influenza B, *Mycoplasma pneumoniae* or infection due to herpes simplex type 1 or herpes simplex type 2
Neutrophilic dermatoses	Sweet's syndrome	Inflammatory syndrome associated most frequently with acute leukemia/myelodysplastic syndromes but also with other conditions
	Pyoderma gangrenosum	Most frequent association is with rheumatoid arthritis and inflammatory bowel disease
Reactive inflammatory syndromes (sometimes postinfectious)	Rheumatic fever Postinfectious reactive arthritis	Group A streptococci Enterocolitic pathogens or genitourinary infections Also due to *Mycobacterium tuberculosis* Poststreptococcal (must be distinguished from rheumatic fever)

TABLE 13.1 Common Noninfectious Inflammatory Syndromes that May Mimic Infectious Diseases[a] (cont.)

Category	Description	Core concepts
Malignancies	Hematologic malignancies	Acute leukemia including hairy cell leukemia and HTLV-related adult T-cell leukemia/lymphoma Lymphomas (Hodgkin's and non-Hodgkin's)
	Solid-organ malignancies	Renal cell carcinoma Hepatocarcinoma Myxoma Glioblastoma multiforme Ovarian carcinoma
Nonbacterial thrombotic endocarditis	Also termed marantic or cachectic (Libman–Sacks endocarditis when it is associated with SLE)	Often embolic and may cause associated-fever
Crystal-induced arthropathies	Monosodium urate	Gout
	Calcium pyrophosphate	Pseudogout
	Calcium oxalate	Oxalosis, vitamin deficiencies, or excess ingestion of particular foods
	Apatite-induced arthropathies	Calcified periarticular lesions (eg, Milwaukee shoulder syndrome)
Autoimmune/ autoinflam- matory	Rheumatoid arthritis	Often presenting as arthralgias, or polyarthritis with undifferentiated fever
	Inflammatory bowel disease	Initial presentation varies but it may potentially be associated with extra-intestinal manifestations (pyoderma gangrenosum, uveitis, spondyloarthropathy, and others)
Autoinflamma- tory periodic febrile syn- dromes	Recurrent hereditary fever syndromes are often associated with different clinical manifestations (some have been associated with monogenic mutations of genes involved in the innate immune response)	FMF (familial Mediterranean fever charac- terized by peritonitits, arthritis, pleuritis) TRAPS (TNF receptor-associated periodic syndrome) PAPA (pyogenic arthritis, pyoderma gangrenosum, and acne) PFAPA (periodic fever, aphtous stomatitis, pharyngitis, and adenitis syndrome) AOSD (adult onset Still's disease – characterized by fever, salmon- colored evanescent rash, hyperferritinemia) Schnitzler's syndrome (urticarial rash, IgM or IgG paraproteinemia, in individuals above 50 years of age) CAPS (cold-induced urticarial rash, arthralgias, conjunctivitis) CANDLE (atypical neutrophilic dermatosis and lypodystrophy) DITRA (generalized pustular psoriasis and general malaise)

(Continued)

TABLE 13.1 Common Noninfectious Inflammatory Syndromes that May Mimic Infectious Diseases[a] (cont.)

Category	Description	Core concepts
Antiphospholipid syndrome	Sometimes when it present as "catastrophic" it may mimic sepsis, heparin-induced thrombocytopenia, thrombotic microangiopathies	Hughes syndrome characterized by both arterial and venous thrombosis and miscarriages due to the presence of antibodies against antiphospholipid molecules including the anticardiolipin antibodies and the lupus anticoagulant and targeted specifically against the beta-2-glycoprotein I and to prothrombin
Miscellaneous	Systemic histiocytosis Systemic mastocytosis Carcinoid syndrome Thyroid storm	Occasionally, a patient with thyroid storm may be initially confused as septic or vice versa; (particularly, when it manifests with elevated transaminases, atrial fibrillation with rapid ventricular response leading to hemodynamic instability and/or respiratory failure

[a]Including some malignancies that cause fever likely due to production of cytokines that raise the hypothalamic set point causing fever and that often respond to naproxen.
[b]Giant cell arteritis needs to be distinguished from trigeminal herpes zoster, trigeminal neuralgia, dental abscess/tumor, bisphosphonate related osteonecrosis of the jaw, temporomandibular joint disease, retinal vascular accident, and nonarteritic anterior ischemic optic neuropathy (eg, severe anemia). However, there is increasing evidence that temporal arteritis, at least in some cases, can be elicited by Varicella–Zoster virus affecting temporal vasculature (Powel DR 2nd, Patel S, Franco-Paredes C. Varicella-Zoster Virus vasculopathy: the growing association between herpes zoster and strokes. Am J Med Sci 2015;350(3):243–245).

TABLE 13.2 Clinical Spectrum and Differential Diagnosis of the Neutrophilic Dermatoses

Category	Description	Core concepts
Sweet syndrome[a] Tender erythematous skin lesions (papules, nodules and plaques) associated with highly-elevated and recurrent fever. Skin biopsy demonstrates Neutrophilic infiltration. Respond to corticosteroids but more than 30% have recurrences	Classical Sweet's syndrome	Usually women between 30–50 years, a preceding upper respiratory infection or associated with inflammatory bowel disease or pregnancy
	Malignancy-associated Sweet's syndrome (MASS)	Most commonly associated with acute myelogenous leukemia or myelodysplastic syndrome Solid tumors: genitourinary organs, breast, and gastrointestinal tract malignancies
	Drug-induced Sweet's syndrome	Granulocyte-colony stimulating factor Trimethoprim-sulfametoxazole

TABLE 13.2 Clinical Spectrum and Differential Diagnosis of the Neutrophilic Dermatoses (*cont.*)

Category	Description	Core concepts
Pyoderma gangrenosum[b] Ulcerative disorder of the skin that can cause severe pain, disfigurement. The borders of the the ulcers are well defined and usually blue color, undermined borders, and often serpiginous configuration. Treatment requires corticosteroids and often other immunosuppressive drugs	Four Types: Classic Ulcerative (Crohn's disease, rheumatoid arthritis) Bullous (acute leukemia) Pustular (acute leukemia/ myelodysplastic syndromes) Vegetative (atypical granulomatosis with polyangiitis)	Around 50% of patients have associated conditions. Most commonly associated with inflammatory bowel disease (Crohn's disease or ulcerative colitis) followed by monoclonal gammopathy, myeloproliferative disorders, hematologic malignancy, Behcet's disease, systemic lupus erythematosus, pregnancy, and Takayasu's arteritis). There are drug related forms: granulocyte stimulating factors, isotretinoin and infections such as HIV, and viral hepatitis C (HCV) Diagnosis is established by the presence of associated conditions and the exclusion of other causes of cutaneous ulcers through biopsy but most importantly clinical observation
Other neutrophilic dermatoses Erythema elevatum diutinum	Leukocytoclastic vasculitis symmetric plaques and nodules	See Table 13.5
Subcorneal pustular dermatosis	Primary lesion is a small sterile pustule arising on normal skin or with a slightly erythematous base that coalesce to form annular or serpiginous patterns	Occurs mainly in women from 40 to 70 years due to an abnormal cytokine response
Rheumatoid neutrophilic dermatitis	Similar cutaneous lesions to pyoderma gangrenosum	It may occur in patients with advanced rheumatoid arthritis

(Continued)

TABLE 13.2 Clinical Spectrum and Differential Diagnosis of the Neutrophilic Dermatoses (*cont.*)

Category	Description	Core concepts
Neutrophilic panniculitis	Painful inflammatory, subcutaneous nodules on the limbs associated with fever, arthralgia, and fatigue	Histopathologically there are lobar panniculitis and it is associated with Sweet's syndrome and pyoderma gangrenosum
Aseptic abscess	Inflammatory condition characterized by deep, sterile and well defined collections of polymorphonuclear cells with pain, high-grade fever and leucocytosis	It is closely related to Sweet's syndrome and pyoderma gangrenosum but it manifests with relapsing subcutaneous painful nodules

[a]Cohen PR. Sweet's syndrome – a comprehensive review of an acute febrile neutrophilic dermatosis. Orphanet J Rare Dis 2007;**2**:34.
[b]Miller J, Yentzer BA, Clark A, Jorizzo JL, Feldman SR. Pyoderma gangrenosum: a review and update on new therapies. J Am Acad Dermatol 2010;**62**:646–654; Rosmaninho A, Carvalho S, Lobo I. Neutrophilic dermatoses revisited. EMJ Dermatol 2014;**2**:77–85.

TABLE 13.3 Clinical Spectrum and Differential Diagnosis of Eosinophilic Skin Diseases[a]

Category	Description	Core concepts
Eosinophilic cellulitis (Well's syndrome)	Mostly presenting in adults with the sudden appearance of multiple or single well circumscribed and large tender erythema and plaques that may have annular configuration	Triggering factors include arthropod bites, viral or bacterial infections, drugs, or vaccines. Some associated diseases include haematological malignancies, chronic myeloid leukemia (CML), Churg–Strauss syndrome, renal cell and colon carcinomas; and also associated with the hypereosinophilic syndrome[b]
Eosinophilic pustular Folliculitis (Ofuji's disease)	Also termed eosinophilic folliculitis and it is a non-infectious inflammatory dermatosis with recurrent episodes of pruritic follicular papules and pustules	Often seen in patients with HIV/AIDS or in some malignancies. May occur or worsen as immune-reconstitution syndrome. Responds to indomethacin

TABLE 13.3 Clinical Spectrum and Differential Diagnosis of Eosinophilic Skin Diseases[a] (*cont.*)

Category	Description	Core concepts
Eosinophilic fasciitis (Schulman disease)	Characterized by symmetrical painful swelling with progressive induration and thickening of the skin and soft tissues of the distal extremities	Scleroderma-like induration with peripheral eosinophilia. Associated with drugs, such as natalizumab, influenza vaccination, simvastatin, phenytoin, subcutaneous administration of heparin, atorvastatin. Also associated with hematologic malignancies in 10% of cases (aplastic anemia, myelomonocytic leukemia, multiple myeloma, and chronic eosinophilic leukemia), and paroxysmal nocturnal hemoglobinuria Magnetic resonance imaging of the affected area and skin biopsy to the muscle assist in confirming the diagnosis
Recurrent cutaneous eosinophlic vasculitis	Recurrent cutaneous necrotizing vasculitis with multiple annular urticarial plaques, angioedema, palpable purpura or hemorrhagic vesicular lesions	Associated with some retroperitoneal fibrosis and likely associated with IgG4-related disease
Granuloma faciale	Manifests as a solitary reddish-violaceous plaque on the face. Histological changes with a Grenz zone (uninvolved dermis)	Affects middle-aged men and more frequently white men. Responds to tacrolimus and laser therapy. Differential diagnosis is mainly with erythema elevatum diutinum, sarcoidosis, discoid lupus and cutaneous tuberculosis
Pemphigus herpetiformis	Resembles dermatitis herpetiformis	
Bullous pemphigoid	Autoimmune subepidermal bullous disease affecting elderly individuals	Subepidermal blisters with eosinophilic infiltration affecting dermal–epidermal junction

(*Continued*)

TABLE 13.3 Clinical Spectrum and Differential Diagnosis of Eosinophilic Skin Diseases[a] (cont.)

Category	Description	Core concepts
Eosinophilic granulomatosis with polyangiitis (Churg–Strauss syndrome)	Characterized as a necrotizing vasculitis with eosinophilic infiltration of medium and small-size vessels	Affects middle aged individuals with a history of asthma and sometimes during tapering of corticosteroids
Hypereosinophilic syndromes	Affects multiple organs with associated persistent peripheral hypereosinopilia	Frequently involves the skin
Episodic angioedema with eosinophilia	Gleich's syndrome characterized by recurrent angioedema, itchy urticarial and weight gain	Presence of eosinophilic infiltrates in the skin, marked blood eosinophilia and elevated IgM levels
Eosinophilic lymphofolliculosis of the skin	Kimura's disease characterized by deep subcutaneous masses involving primarily the head and neck region	Associated regional lymphadenopathy and salivary gland involvement with eosinophilic infiltration and elevated IgE levels
Epitheloid hemangioma	Angiolymphoid hyperplasia with eosinophilia	Mutiple red to brown firm papules and nodules occurring in the head and neck region with a predilection for the peri-auricular area in adults

[a]There is a broad spectrum of skin disease that are characterized by eosinophil infiltration and/or degranulation in skin lesions, and that maybe associated or not with systemic eosinophilia (Long H, Zhang G, Wang L, Lui Q. Eosinophilic skin diseases: a comprehensive review. Clinic Rev Allerg Immunol 2015;doi 10.1007/s12016-015-8485-8).
[b]A count of more than 1,500 eosinophils per microliter of blood is considered hypereosinophilia.

TABLE 13.4 Pulmonary and Eosinophilia Syndromes

Category	Description	Core concepts
Eosinophilic Pneumonias (usually not associated with peripheral eosinophilia)	Acute eosinophilic pneumonia	Rapid onset of respiratory symptoms (usually within a week. Eosinophilic count in bronchoalveolar lavage >25%[a]
	Chronic eosinophilic pneumonia	Subacute course with high. Eosinophilic count in bronchoalveolar lavage >25%

TABLE 13.4 Pulmonary and Eosinophilia Syndromes (*cont.*)

Category	Description	Core concepts
Eosinophilic granulomatosis with polyangiitis (Churg–Strauss syndrome)	Affects middle-aged individuals with a history of asthma and sometimes during tapering of corticosteroids	Necrotizing vasculitis with eosinophilic infiltration of lung of medium-size and small-size vessels in the lungs. Eosinophilic count in bronchoalveolar lavage >25%
Allergic bronchopulmonary aspergillosis (ABPA)	Affects patients with a history of asthma. It is likely a hypersensitivity reaction to *Aspergillus* colonizing the airways without evidence of pulmonary parenchymal invasion	Worsening asthma symptoms with expectoration of brownish collections of mucus and central bronchiectasis
Hypersensitivity Pneumonitis	Not associated with peripheral eosinophilia but with persistent pulmonary infiltrates, cough, and worsening respiratory failure	Responds to steroids, sometimes many family members living in the same household or exposed to the same environments may occur at the same time. Obtaining exposure history is crucial
Drug related	Patients may have peripheral eosinophilia and high eosinophil counts in bronchoalveolar lavage	Nitrofurantoin (often the cause of patients on chronic suppressive dosing for recurrent urinary tract infections in the elderly and nursing home residents) Sulfa drugs Amiodarone NSAIDs Minocycline Phenytoin
Parasitic Infections	Transpulmonary transit of larval parasitic forms Parenchymal Disease/ invasion	*Ascaris lumbricoides, Ancylostoma duodenale, Necator americanus, Strongyloides stercolaris Paragonimus westermani or Paragonimus pacificus*

(Continued)

TABLE 13.4 Pulmonary and Eosinophilia Syndromes (*cont.*)

Category	Description	Core concepts
Hypersensitivity reaction to Filarial Infection (*Wuchereria bancrofti* and *Brugia malayi*)	Tropical pulmonary eosinophilia (immune reaction to the filarial antigen γ-glutamil transpeptidase)	Represents a hypersensitivity reaction localized to the lung in individuals most frequently of the Indian subcontinent ancestry and with a history of asthma or chronic lung disease. Eosinophilic count in bronchoalveolar lavage >25%
	Disseminated disease[b]	Visceral larva migrans due to *Toxocara cati* or *Toxocara canis*
		Disseminated strongyloidiasis or hyperinfection syndrome in immunocompromised hosts
Hypereosinophilic syndromes (when no other parasitic, neoplastic of inflammatory condition hypereosinophlia and organ damage)	Chronic eosinophilic leukemia Lymphocytic hypereosinophilia Myeloproliferative hypereosinophilia	In most of these condition there is lung involvement which can range from bronchial hyperreactivity, pulmonary infiltrates, peripheral eosinophilia, and even pulmonary fibrosis with restrictive a restrictive pattern in association with involvement of other organs

[a]There is often moderate eosinophil count elevation (<25%) in patients with drug-induced pneumonitis, fungal pneumonias, in some forms of idiopathic pulmonary fibrosis, sarcoidosis, and in those with Langerhans cell histiocytosis.
[b]Chronic schistosomiasis rarely produces pulmonary infiltrates since it involves mainly the pulmonary vasculature leading to pulmonary hypertension.

TABLE 13.5 Differential Diagnosis of Cutaneous Erythema Syndromes

Category	Description	Core concepts
Erythema nodosum	Red nodules with inflammation of fat cells under the skin (lobar panniculitis), most commonly presenting as tender red nodules on the extensor surfaces of the lower extremities; it is considered an immunologic response to a variety of eliciting factors. There is an association with HLA-B27	Associations: Idiopathic, sarcoidosis (Löfgren's syndrome)[a], group A streptococci pharyngitis, upper viral respiratory infections, tuberculosis, coccidiodomycosis, *Salmonella, Yersinia, Campylobacter, hepatitis B virus, Mycoplasma pneumoniae, Brucella mellitensis, Chlamydia pneumoniae, Chlamydia trachomatis* Drug related: beta-lactam antibiotics, sulfa drugs, oral contraceptives), inflammatory bowel disease, Behcet's syndrome, Sweet's syndrome, and hematologic malignancies
Erythema induratum (Bazin's erythema)	Similar to erythema nodosum it is a nodular vasculitis and causes panniculitis but involving a different pattern (septolobular pattern with neutrophilic vasculitis). It frequently involves the posterior aspect of the lower extremities. Nodules evolve over several weeks often developing ulceration and, sometimes, drainage	Frequent association with exposure to *Mycobacterium tuberculosis*. However, there are many reports of *Nocardia, Pseudomonas,* and *Fusarium* and rarely in chronic viral hepatitis C. Non-infectious conditions associated with erythema induratum include Crohn's disease, rheumatoid arthritis, and chronic lymphocytic leukemia
Erythema marginatum	Associated with rheumatic fever and often identified in the upper and lower extremities. It appears as a non-tender pink or red macules or papules which spread centripetally often in a circular shape. As the lesions progressed and coalesce the borders become raised and erythematous with a clear centre.	Present in rheumatic fever, particularly in children with carditis. The lesions can fade and reappear within a few hours and this pattern may last for a few weeks or months

(Continued)

TABLE 13.5 Differential Diagnosis of Cutaneous Erythema Syndromes (cont.)

Category	Description	Core concepts
Erythema elevatum diutinum	Deposition of immune complexes secondary to streptococcal infections, hematologic malignancies, or autoimmune diseases	Nodular lesions and plaques involving symmetrically extensor surfaces hands, feet, elbows, knees or buttocks. Immune complex deposition leading to a leukocytoclastic vasculitis occurring in individuals above 50 years of age. Older lesions have yellow brown coloration that resembles xanthomas of cholesterol
Erythema multi-forme[b]	Acute immune-mediated condition that may affect the skin and mucosae (erythema minor is defined as no mucosal involvement)	There are distinctive annular and target like lesions of the skin. Most episodes are self-limiting but could be potentially recurrent and it affects all age groups. It is most frequently associated to drugs (beta-lactam antibiotics, sulfa drugs, anticonvulsants such as valproate or phenytoin and other drugs) Also associated with genital or oral herpes associated with herpes simplex type 1 and type 2, and infection due to *Mycoplasma pneumoniae*, and influenza B[c]

[a]*Common sarcoidosis syndromes include: Löfgren's syndrome (erythema nodosum, bilateral hilar adenopathy, arthritis/arthralgias occurring in 35% of cases and carries a good response to steroids and prognosis); Heerfordt–Waldenstrom syndrome (fever, parotid enlargement, anterior uveitis, facial nerve palsy, papilledema, lethargy, meningismus in some cases and common in some Caribbean populations); Mikulic's syndrome (bilateral enlargement of the parotid, submandibular, sublingual, and lacrimal glands); and Darier–Roussy syndrome (multiple subcutaneous nontender nodules).*
[b]*Erythema multiforme is a distinct clinical entity from Stevens–Johnson(SJS)/toxic epidermic necrolysis (TEN) spectrum of disease and should not be clinically confused.*
[c]*There is considerable evidence that the herpes viruses modulate the inflammatory response in many clinical situations including drug-reaction. For example, drug reaction eosinophilic system syndrome has been associated with human herpes virus-6 (HHV-6), Epstein–Barr virus causing infectious mononucleosis causing a drug-reaction to beta-lactam antibiotics, and it is likely that erythema multiforme is a disease caused by immunomodulation caused by herpes simplex viruses in susceptible patients receiving a drug that elicits the reaction. Interestingly, the recurrent nature of erythema multiforme also mimics the pattern of reactivation of herpes simplex viruses type 1 and type 2.*

REFERENCES

1. McGonalge D, McDermott MF. A proposed classification of the immunological diseases. *PLoS Med* 2006;**3**(8):e297.
2. Kallinich T, Gattorno M, Grattan CE, de Koning HA, Traidl Hoffmann C, Feist T, et al. Unexplained recurrent fever: when is autoinflammation the explanation? *Allergy* 2013;**68**:285–96.
3. Ravelli A, Davi S, Minoia F, Martini A, Cron RQ. Macrophage activation syndrome. *Hematol Oncol Clin N Am* 2015;**11**(9):1043–53.
4. Rouphael NG, Talati NJ, Vaughan C, Cunningham K, Moreira R, Gould C. Infections associated with haemophagocytic syndrome. *Lancet Infect Dis* 2007;**7**:814–22.
5. George JN, Nester CN. Syndromes of thrombotic microangiopathy. *N Engl. J Med* 2014;**371**(7):654–66.
6. Kanisawa T, Zen Y, Pillai S, Stone JH. IgG4-related disease. *Lancet* 2015;**385**(9976):1460–71.
7. Horowitz HW. Fever of unknown origin or fever of too many origins? *N Engl. J Med* 2013;**368**(3):197–9.
8. Cunha BA, Lortholary O, Cunha CB. Fever of unknown origin: a clinical approach. *Am J Med* 2015;**128**:1138.e1–1138.e15.

Chapter 14

Syndromes in Travel and Tropical Medicine

DIAGNOSTIC APPROACH TO TRAVEL AND TROPICAL MEDICINE SYNDROMES

Particular groups of travelers are considered at higher risk for illness. Travelers visiting friends and relatives are often less likely to seek pre-travel advice, obtain vaccinations, or take antimalarial prophylaxis.[1–3] Adventure travelers and people visiting friends and relatives are at increased risk for becoming ill, in part because of increased exposure to pathogens. Similarly, people with underlying immunocompromised status may be at increased risk of illness, as well as atypical manifestations of disease.[4]

In addition to the clinical picture, the pretravel preparation and exposure histories form the basis of the differential diagnosis. The immunization history will often rule out particular entities such as hepatitis A, hepatitis B, yellow fever, meningococcal meningitis, and Japanese encephalitis in those who have been immunized. On the other hand, a history of typhoid immunization does not rule out infection since the vaccine is only 70% effective.[5–6] A history of malaria chemoprophylaxis should include the name of drug, dose, patient adherence to the regimen, and whether the patient is still on the drug on return. It is extremely rare for a traveler to develop *Plasmodium falciparum* malaria if the antimalarial drug, dose and adherence are appropriate to national guidelines.

CLINICAL SYNDROMES IN TRAVEL AND TROPICAL MEDICINE

In the practice of travel medicine, narrowing the differential diagnosis of an illness in the returned traveler is achieved by identifying the likely causative cause by (1) obtaining a detailed pretravel and travel history including exact arrival and departure dates; (2) assessing the constellation of signs and symptoms, including incubation periods (Table 14.1), and (3) taking a history of specific exposures[7–10] (Table 14.2). Most travelers infected abroad become ill within 12 weeks after returning to the United States. However, some infections may not cause symptoms for as long as 6–12 months or more after exposure. When an infectious disease is suspected, calculating an approximate incubation period is a useful step in ruling out possible causes.[10–13] For example, fever beginning

Core Concepts in Clinical Infectious Diseases (CCCID). http://dx.doi.org/10.1016/B978-0-12-804423-0.00014-7

173

TABLE 14.1 Clinical Febrile Syndromes in Returned Travelers[a]

Incubation period	Clinical syndrome[b]	Etiologies
<2 weeks	Undifferentiated fever	Malaria, dengue, chikungunya, spotted group rickettsiae, acute HIV, Campylobacter, salmonellosis, enteric fever East African trypanosomiasis, leptospirosis, relapsing fever
	Fever and coagulopathy	Meningococcemia, leptospirosis, and other bacterial pathogens associated with coagulopathy, malaria, viral hemorrhagic fevers (ie, Lassa fever, Ebola)
	Fever and central nervous system syndrome	Malaria, typhoid fever, rickettsial typus (epidemic caused by *Rickettsia Prowazecki*), meningococcal meningitis, rabies, arboviral encephalitis, East African trypanosomiasis, cosmopolitan causes of encephalitis or meningitis angiostrongyloidiasis, rabies
	Fever and pulmonary syndrome	Influenza, community-acquired pneumonia (typical and atypical pathogens), acute histoplasmosis, acute coccidiodomycosis, Q fever, SARS
	Fever and skin rash	Viral exanthems (rubella, varicella, mumps, human herpesvirus-6), dengue, spotted or typhus group rickettsiosis, enteric fever, parvovirus B19
2–6 Weeks	Various syndromes (fever with pulmonary, cutaneous, neurologic, or other sites)	Malaria, tuberculosis, hepatitis A, hepatitis B, hepatitis E, visceral leishmaniasis, acute schistosomiasis, amebic liver abscess, leptospirosis, African trypanosomiasis, viral hemorrhagic fevers, Q fever, acute American trypanosomiasis, typhoid fever
>6 Weeks	Other syndromes (fever with pulmonary, cutaneous, neurologic, or other sites)	Malaria, tuberculosis, hepatitis B, hepatitis E, visceral leishmaniasis, filariasis, onchocerciasis, schistosomiasis, amebic liver abscess, chronic mycoses, African trypanosomiasis, and rabies

[a]*Franco-Paredes C, Keystone J. Fever in the returned traveler. In: Empiric (www.antimicrobe.org). Yu VL, et al, editors. ESun Technologies, Pittsburgh, PA, 2011.*
[b]*Franco-Paredes C, Hochberg N. General Approach to the returned traveler. In: Kozarksy P, Magill A, Shlim D, editors. Yellow Book: Health Information for Travelers 2011–2012, Centers for Disease Control and Prevention, Elsevier Ltd, 2011.*

TABLE 14.2 History of Exposures and Corresponding Syndrome or Disease[a]

Exposure	Clinical syndrome or specific disease
Ill persons	Viral hepatitis, enteric fever, influenza, viral hemorrhagic fever (Lassa, Ebola), tuberculosis
Animals	Rabies, Q fever, plague, tularemia, borreliosis, histoplasmosis (caves), anthrax
Arthropod bites Mosquitoes Ticks	Malaria, dengue, chikungunya, zika Typhus, borreliosis, relapsing fever, scrub typhus
Reduviid bugs Tse tse flies	Acute Chagas disease African trypanosomiasis (Human African Trypanosomiasis – HAT)
Food (raw, undercooked meat)	Hepatitis A or hepatitis E, bacterial gastroenteritis, trichinosis, non-typhoidal salmonellosis (*Salmonella* Typhimurium), enteric fever
Food (unpasteurized dairy) Raw fish (ceviche or sashimi)	Listeriosis, brucellosis, bovine TB Anisakiasis, ghanthostomiasis
Fresh water	Schistosomiasis, leptospirosis, *Mycobacterium marinum*
Secretions of nonhuman primates	Herpes B virus
Estuary water	*Vibrio cholera* *Vibrio vulnificus* (blistering cellulitis with sepsis in patients with excess iron including those with chronic liver disease) *Aeromonas hydrophila* (necrotizing fasciitis or rapidly progressive cellulitis)
Sexual contact, tattoing, piercing	Syphilis, gonococcemia, HIV, hepatitis B,C, HTVL-1
History of travel to some sites in Southeast Asia[b]	Invasive *Klebsiella pneumoniae* syndrome associated with bacteremia, liver abscess, and metastatic infection (endophtalmitis)[b]
History of travel to some sites in Southeast Asia (Northeastern Thailand, Malaysia, Singapore, Vietnam, Cambodia and Laos); and Northern Australia[c]	Community-acquired sepsis due to *Burkholderia pseudomallei*

[a]*Franco-Paredes C, Keystone J. Fever in the returned traveler. In: Empiric (www.antimicrobe.org). Yu VL, et al, editors. ESun Technologies, Pittsburgh, PA, 2011.*
[b]*Nadasy KA, Domiati-Saad R, Tribble MA. Invasive* Klebsiella pneumoniae *syndrome in North America. Clin Infect Dis 2007;**45**:e25–e28.*
[c]*Wiersinga WJ, Currie BJ, Peacock SJ. Melioidosis. N Engl. J Med 2012;**367**(11):1035–1044.*

≥3 weeks after return substantially reduces the probability of dengue, rickettsial infections, and viral hemorrhagic fevers in the differential diagnosis. Late-appearing illnesses include chronic forms of Chagas disease, cutaneous and mucocutaneous leishmaniasis, chronic forms of brucellosis, reactivation of tuberculosis from travel-acquired latent tuberculosis infection, malaria, sequelae of schistosomiasis, and reactivation of chronic systemic mycoses, such as paracoccidioidomycosis or coccidioidomycosis.[11–24]

The exposure history is crucial to the formulation of a differential diagnosis. Eliciting a detailed history of the specific locales visited, the timing of travel relative to the onset of symptoms, the exact arrival and departure dates, and specific risk behavior is essential in determining potential exposure to infectious pathogens and likely incubation period. As noted in Table 14.2 the exposure history should include a history of contact with animals (including bites), new sexual partners, freshwater, insects (especially ticks and tsetse flies), medical equipment (needles, blood transfusions), and ill persons. Also, a history of ingestion of unpasteurized dairy products or uncooked meat as well as an occupational history might be important for the differential diagnosis.[25] It is important to remember that particular groups of travelers are considered at higher risk of developing illness after returning to their place of residence. Adventure travelers and those persons visiting friends and relatives overseas are at greatest risk for becoming ill, in part because of increased exposure to pathogens. Also, those visiting friends and relatives (VFRs) are less likely to seek pretravel advice, to take antimalarial prophylaxis, and to receive travel-related vaccinations.[1,2,4] The most frequent health problems in ill returned travelers are persistent gastrointestinal illness (10%), skin lesions or rashes (8%), respiratory infections (5–13%, depending on season of travel), and fever (up to 3%).[26] In terms of clinical severity, most travel-related illnesses are mild, but between 1–5% of travelers become sick enough to seek medical care either during or after travel. Thus, a travel history, particularly travel within the previous 6 months, should be part of the routine medical history in every ill patient, especially in those with fever.

FEVER AND TRAVEL

The clinical approach of a febrile traveler recently returned from resource-poor settings requires detailed knowledge of the patient's pretravel preparation, travel itinerary, and exposure history. In many cases, the etiology of the febrile illness will not have a destination-related cause and often the illness will be self-limited without a diagnosis being confirmed. However, the workup-of such patients should always be considered a medical emergency and, where indicated, "malaria until proven otherwise". Infectious disease or tropical medicine specialists should be consulted when such expertise is required (Table 14.3). For diagnostic purposes, fevers may be viewed as acute, subacute, or chronic, and with or without localizing signs. The most frequent health problems in ill

TABLE 14.3 Laboratory and Imaging Studies to Consider in a Returned Traveler Presenting with a Febrile Syndrome[a]

Core laboratory testing	Complete blood count with manual differential Comprehensive metabolic panel Urianalysis Thin and thick peripheral blood smear for detection of malaria parasites Malaria testing (rapid testing, molecular nucleic acid assays) Stool culture and/or ova and parasites in stools X 3 Chest radiograph
Additional more specific testing[b]	Rickettsial serology *Schistosoma* serology *Leptospira* serology Viral hepatitis serologies HIV ELISA and/or HIV RNA viral load Skin biopsy CT scanning or MRI depending on the clinical syndrome

[a]*Franco-Paredes C, Keystone J. Fever in the returned traveler. In: Empiric (www.antimicrobe.org). Yu VL, et al., editors. ESun Technologies, Pittsburgh, PA, 2014.*
[b]*Franco-Paredes C, Hochberg N. General approach to the returned traveler. In: Kozarsky P, Magill A, Shlim D, editors. Yellow Book: Health Information for Travelers 2011–2012, Centers for Disease Control and Prevention, Elsevier Ltd, 2011.*

returned travelers are persistent gastrointestinal illness, 10% cutaneous lesions, 8%; respiratory infections, 5–13% (depending on season of travel); and fever in up to 3%. Although gastrointestinal upset is the most frequent problem, febrile illness is the most serious since the infection may be life threatening to the patient (malaria or meningococcal meningitis) or a pose a serious public health hazard (tuberculosis, measles, or viral hemorrhagic fevers). Different reports by the Geosentinel travel and tropical medical clinics on six continents has shown significant regional differences in terms of morbidity in various syndromic categories in relation to place of exposure among ill returned travelers. For example, dermatologic problems were among the most important diagnosis among those travelers returning from the Caribbean or Central or South America, whereas the diagnosis of acute diarrheal illness was more common for those travelers returning from South Central Asia. Malaria was identified as one of the three most frequent causes of systemic febrile illness among travelers from any region. Besides malaria, travelers returning from Southern Africa were diagnosed with a rickettsial infection, primarily tick-borne spotted fever. Dengue fever or chikungunya are rarely seen in travelers from Africa but common in those returned from Southeast Asia and the Caribbean.

Most travelers infected abroad become ill within 12 weeks after returning to the United States. However, some diseases, such as malaria, may not cause symptoms for as long as 6–12 months after exposure. If travelers become ill after they return home, even many months after travel, they should be advised to tell their physician where and when they have traveled. Fever patterns are sometimes helpful in dissecting febrile-illnesses in travelers. Continuous fever pattern may indicate the possibility of enteric fever or typhus; remittent fever may indicate tuberculosis, African trypanosomiasis; intermittent fever may be due to malaria or tuberculosis; and relapsing fever may be due to louse-borne *Borrelia recurrentis* or *Borrelia duttoni* tick-borne infection or malaria. The fever pattern associated with *falciparum* and *knowlesi* malaria rarely display periodicity. A classic alternate day or every third day fever is virtually pathognomonic for malaria, the former *P. vivax* and the latter *P. malariae*. In particular, fever in a returned traveler from a malarious area should be considered to be malaria until proven otherwise and a medical emergency; the diagnosis of malaria should be evaluated urgently by appropriate laboratory tests and qualified personnel.[26–28]

GASTROINTESTINAL DISEASE AND TRAVEL

Acute bacterial gastroenteritis and parasitic diarrhea, caused mostly by *Giardia*, are overall the most common conditions reported by travelers. Parasitic diarrhea may often present as intermittent diarrhea, nausea, headache, and fatigue but may also present with postprandial rapid expulsions of loose stool.

Persistent gastrointestinal illness in returned travelers is often caused by postinfectious irritable bowel syndrome and postinfectious lactose intolerance after an episode of travelers' diarrhea. However, sometimes an infectious pathogen may uncover or trigger an underlying or previously subclinical condition such as celiac sprue or inflammatory bowel disease. Additionally, intestinal parasitic infections are uncommon causes of persistent diarrhea, although infections including *Giardia lamblia* and *Cyclospora cayetanensis* are often treated on the basis of clinical findings without laboratory confirmation. A wide variety of gastrointestinal/abdominal syndromes may present in a traveler (Table 14.4).[10,13]

DERMATOLOGIC CONDITIONS AND TRAVEL

Dermatologic conditions are a very common reason for posttravel consultation. Most post-travel skin ailments reported are insect bites, cutaneous larva migrans, myiasis, pyoderma, scabies, and viral exanthems (Table 14.5).[13,27]

EOSINOPHILIA AND TRAVEL

Table 14.6 depicts causes of eosinophilia in travelers. It is important to note that most often eosinophilia in a returning traveler usually indicates a parasitic infection. Diagnoses to be considered in travelers with moderate to marked eosinophilia (>1000 eosinophils/mm^3) include acute schistosomiasis or strongyloidiasis, toxocariasis, acute trichinellosis, lymphatic filariasis, loiasis, onchocerciasis, tropical pulmonary eosinophilia, fascioliasis, gnathostomiasis,

TABLE 14.4 Common Gastrointestinal Syndromes in Travelers[a]

Category	Etiology
Acute diarrheal	Gastroenteritis (watery diarrhea with vomiting): Enterotoxigenic *E. Coli, Campylobacter jejuni, Shigella*, nontyphoidal salmonellosis Inflammatory/invasive/dysentery (*Shigella dysenteriae, Entamoeba histolytica*) Secretory-toxin mediated (*Vibrio cholera* 01)
Dysphagia	Esophageal candidiasis Achalasia-like illness due to *Trypanosoma cruzi*
Peptic ulcer disease	*Helicobacter pylori*
Gastrointestinal bleeding	Esophageal varices due to chronic *Schistosoma mansoni* infection Cirrhosis with portal hypertension due to chronic hepatitis B or C
Enteric fever	*Salmonella* Typhi *Salmonella* Paratyphi A/B/C
Persistent infection	*Giardia lamblia* Whipple's disease (associated with neurological, fever of unknown origin, mesenteric lymphadenopathy, and arthralgias) Tropical sprue *Entamoeba histolytica* *Cyclospora cayetanensis*
Abdominal mass	Hepatocarcinoma due to hepatitis B or cirrhosis caused by hepatitis B or C
Perforation peritonitis	Enteric fever (usually untreated between second and third week of illness) Gastrointestinal tuberculosis (usually caused by *Mycobacterium bovis*)
Severe abdominal pain	*Angyostrongyloides costaricensis*[b] *Fasciola hepatica* Soil-transmitted helminths (Strongyloidiasis, Ascariasis, Trichuriasis)
Oral lesions/ ulcerations	Noma Aphtous stomatitis Disseminated histoplasmosis Mucocutaneous leishmaniasis (*Leishmania braziliensis*) Rhinoscleroma Paracoccidiodomycosis (*Paracoccidiodes brasiliensis*) Crohn's disease
Cholangitis	*Ascaris lumbricoides* invading the biliary tract Clonorchiasis/Opistorchiasis
Abdominal pain and jaundice	Cholangitis Amoebic liver abscess *Fasciola hepatica* Leptospirosis Drug reaction eosinophilic systemic syndrome (DRESS)[c]

(Continued)

TABLE 14.4 Common Gastrointestinal Syndromes in Travelers[a] *(cont.)*

Category	Etiology
Postinfectious Syndromes	Lactose intolerance Irritable bowel syndrome Celiac disease/gluten intolerance Tropical sprue Inflammatory bowel disease

[a]Franco-Paredes C, Hochberg N. General approach to the returned rraveler. In: Kozarksy P, Magill A, Shlim D, editors. Yellow Book: Health Information for Travelers 2011–2012, Centers for Disease Control and Prevention, Elsevier Ltd, 2011.
[b]Angiostrongyloides costaricencis may cause abdominal pain mimicking appendicitis. Sometimes it may mimic a toxic shock syndrome.
[c]DRESS may mimic leptospirosis due to jaundice, renal insufficiency.

TABLE 14.5 Common Cutaneous Syndromes in Travelers[a]

Categories	Etiologies	Core concepts
Eschar	Tick-borne spotted fever rickettsias	*Ricketsia africae* *Ricketsia parkeri*
Maculopapular	Viral exanthems	Measles, HHV-6, parvovirus B19, rubella
	Drug reactions	DRESS
	Rickettsial	Murine typhus, ehrlichiosis
	Mosquito borne	Dengue, chikungunya
Nodular	Prurigo nodularis	Insect bites
	Nodular lymphangitic (spread pattern)	*Mycobacterium marinum* *Nocardia brasiliensis* Sporotricosis *Staphylococcus aureus* Bartonellosis Tularemia Blastomycosis
	Pyogenic folliculitis, carbuncles	*Staphylococcus aureus, Streptococcus* spp.
	Angioedema	Calabar swelling associated with loiasis
	Myiasis	Tumbu fly (*Cordylobia anthrophaga*) in Africa Bot fly (*Dermatobia hominis*) in Central and South America
	Tungiasis	*Tunga penetrans* (sand flea)
Ulcers	Cutaneous leishmaniasis Paracoccidiodomycosis	New and old world strains Central and South America
Macular	Hypopygmented and anesthetic	*M. leprae* (tuberculoid or borderline tuberculoid)

TABLE 14.5 Common Cutaneous Syndromes in Travelers[a] *(cont.)*

Categories	Etiologies	Core concepts
Linear lesions	Cutanea larva migrans	*Ancylostoma braziliense*
	Phytophotodermatitis	Linear hyperpigmentation due to lime juice, mango, or other fruits
	Larva currens	*Strongyloides stercolaris*
Other	Water exposure (cellulitis, blistering cellulitis, nodules)	*M. marinum*
		Erysipelothrix rhusiopathae
		Vibrio vulnificus
		Edwardsiella tarda
		Aeromonas hydrophyla[b]
	Hot tubs	*Pseudomonas aeruginosa*
		Staphylococcus aureus
		Non-tuberculous mycobacteria (*M. chelonei* or *M. fortuitum*)
	Dog bites/Cat bites	*Pasteurella multocida*, HACEK[c]
		Capnocytophaga canimorsus

[a]*Franco-Paredes C, Hochberg N. General approach to the returned traveler. In: Kozarsky P, Magill A, Shlim D, editors. Yellow Book: Health Information for Travelers 2011-2012, Centers for Disease Control and Prevention, Elsevier Ltd, 2011.*
[b]*See chapter: Cutaneous, Subcutaneous, and Deep-Tissue Infections.*
[c]*HACEK refers to gram negative bacilli including* Hemophilus paraprophilus, Actinobacillus actinomycetemcomitans, Cardiobacterium hominis, Eikenella corrodens *and* Kingella.

angiostrongyliasis, and the larval migration of ascariasis, paragonimiasis, and hookworm. Infectious causes of eosinophilia caused by other infectious pathogens include HIV, human T-cell lymphotropic virus type 1, coccidioidomycosis, and allergic bronchopulmonary aspergillosis.[13]

DIAGNOSTIC APPROACH TO COMMON TROPICAL DISEASES

The most frequent tropical causes of fever in the returned traveler are malaria, dengue fever, invasive bacterial gastroenteritis, hepatitis A, enteric fever, and rickettsial infections.[14,21] Nonimmune individuals are particularly susceptible to develop severe malaria due to Plasmodium falciparum and to die from it. On the other hand, immigrants from developing countries who live in malaria-free nations and return home to visit friends and relatives in their place of birth are at much higher risk of acquiring malaria. Indeed, this particular group of travelers has the highest proportion of imported malaria. The majority of VFRs adults does not receive malaria chemoprophylaxis and are not aware that, without repeated exposure, their partial immunity to malaria wanes over time. Their risk is particularly high because they have prolonged stays in their country of origin; and often spends time in high-risk areas without taking any personal protective measures against malaria.

Malaria is the most frequent infectious cause of death in the returned traveler; death may occur within several days of the onset of symptoms. Since all

TABLE 14.6 Common Causes of Eosinophilia in Travelers[a]

Categories	Etiologies	Core concepts
Bacterial	Streptococcal	Resolving scarlet fever Patients with adrenal insufficiency caused by tuberculosis
	Mycobacterium tuberculosis	Miliary tuberculosis (may also present with a leukemoid reaction)
Viral	HIV	
Fungal	Aspergillosis	Allergic bronchopulmonary aspergilosis (ABPA)
	Coccidiodomycosis	Disseminated disease and sometimes during acute phase of infection
Protozoan	*Isosporal belli* *Dientamoeba fragilis* *Sarcocystis*	
Helminthic	Roundworms (Ascariasis, trichinellosis, strongyloidiasis, hookworm, *Capillariasis philippinensis, Capillariasis hepatica*) Trematodes (Clonorchiasis, fascioliasis, fasciolopsiasis, paragonomiasis, schistosomiasis) Cestodes (Echinococcosis) Filarial (Loiasis, onchocerciasis, tropical pulmonary eosinophilia due to *Wuchereria bancrofti*) Visceral larva migrans (Gnathostomiasis, anisakiasis, *Toxocara cati, Toxocara canis, Bayliscaris procyonis*)	Eosinophilia is common with multicellular, helminthic parasites, especially those invading tissues
Drug reaction	Drug Reaction Eosinophilic Systemic Syndrome	May be life-threatening and it is crucial to have a low suspicion threshold

[a]*Franco-Paredes C, Hochberg N. General approach to the returned traveler. In: Kozarksy P, Magill A, Shlim D, editors. Yellow Book: Health Information for Travelers 2011–2012, Centers for Disease Control and Prevention, Elsevier Ltd, 2011.*

prophylactic antimalarial drugs do not prevent the parasite from entering the liver, even individuals who had adhered to appropriate chemoprophylaxis may still acquire the infection.[22,25] Dormant hypnozoites of *P. vivax* or *P. ovale* may be released from the liver into the bloodstream many months or even year after infection occurs. However, 98% of all imported *Plasmodium falciparum* malaria infections, and 74% of *Plasmodium vivax* infections present within 2 months of return. Also, it is important to remember that more than 90% of imported *Plasmodium falciparum* infections originate in sub-Saharan Africa. Malaria symptoms are usually nonspecific and, unless periodic fever occurs, cannot be differentiated from the usual flu-like viral illness. Fever, chills (with or without rigors), headache, and myalgia are most common; dry cough and abdominal pain not infrequently accompany these symptoms. As noted previously, the fever pattern may be helpful, especially for the benign malarias.

Dengue fever also presents with flu-like symptoms, of which the classical features are fever, severe myalgia, headache, retroorbital pain, and a maculo popular rash.[13,16,17] The vast majorities of dengue patients become ill within 7 days of exposure and are afebrile within 7 days of the onset of the illness. Dengue and chikungunya are diagnosed by serology and viral isolation. The infection is most frequently acquired from a day-biting mosquito in SE Asia and the Caribbean, but very rarely in Africa. Chikungunya virus is responsible for an illness that strongly resembles dengue fever with the difference that arthralgia and arthritis replace the myalgia and bone pain of dengue. Older individuals are most likely to suffer from prolonged, disabling, symmetrical, distal polyarthritis. Diagnosis is by serology. Like dengue, it has a short incubation period and is transmitted by a day-biting mosquito. Chikungunya is found primarily in Africa, the Indian subcontinent, Southeast Asia and more recently, the islands of the Indian Ocean and most recently, from the Caribbean.

The classical presentation of enteric fever (typhoid and paratyphoid fevers)[5,13] begins with gradual onset of fever that builds to a crescendo over several days to become a persistent fever, often associated with nonspecific temperature/pulse dissociation. Additional symptoms usually include headache, cough and, unlike nontyphoidal salmonellosis, constipation. Almost any fever pattern can be seen in those with enteric fever; as noted previously, prior immunization does not exclude the diagnosis since the vaccine is only 70% effective. The diagnosis is confirmed by blood cultures that are usually positive during the first week of illness and by stool and urine cultures that become positive during and after the second week of illness.

Tick typhus, due to *Rickettsia africae* is the most frequent cause of fever in a returned traveler from Southern Africa and usually presents with fever, localized tender lymphadenopathy, and a macular or popular rash.[18,19] However, the diagnosis is confirmed clinically by the finding of a tick eschar—a 1–2 cm, black, necrotic lesion with an erythematous margin. The diagnosis may be missed if the patient's skin is not fully examined. Diagnosis is by serology, often utilizing acute and convalescent specimens. Depending upon the exposure history, time course of the illness, and associated signs and symptoms, initial investigations for febrile travelers may include prompt evaluation of peripheral blood smears or a rapid antigen detection method for Plasmodium spp or molecular amplification methods and a complete blood cell count and differential, liver function tests, urinalysis, blood, stool and urine cultures, chest radiography, and specific serologic assays, such as those for the diagnosis of dengue, rickettsial infections, schistosomiasis, leptospirosis, viral hepatitis, HIV etc. (Table 14.3). For this reason, at the initial assessment it is often valuable to keep a serum sample stored for later testing when acute and convalescent serology are needed. Thick and thin blood films or rapid diagnostic antigen testing for malaria should be repeated twice, 12–24 h apart if the initial result is negative.

REFERENCES

1. Angell SY, Cetron MS. Health disparities among travelers visiting friends and relatives abroad. *Ann Intern Med* 2005;**142**:67–72.
2. Angell SY, Behrens RH. Risk assessment and disease prevention in travelers visiting friends and relatives. *Infect Dis Clin North Am* 2005;**19**:67–72.
3. Ansart S, Perez L, Vergely O, Danis M, Bricaire F, Caumes E. Illnesses in travelers returning from the tropics: a prospective study of 622 patients. *J Trav Med* 2005;**12**:312–8.
4. Bacaner N, Stauffer B, Boulware DR, Walker PF, Keystone JS. Travel medicine considerations for North American immigrants visiting friends and relatives. *JAMA* 2004;**291**:2856–64.
5. Basnyat B, Maskey AP, Zimmerman MD, Murdoch DR. Enteric (typhoid) fever in travelers. *Clin Infect Dis* 2005;**15**:1467–72.
6. Bottieau E, Clerinx J, Schrooten W, Van den Enden E, Wouters R, Van Esbroeck M, et al. Etiology and outcome of fever after a stay in the tropics. *Arch Intern Med* 2006;**166**:1642–8.
7. Centers for Disease Control and Prevention. Fatal yellow fever in a traveler returning from Amazonas, Brazil, 2002. *MMWR.* 2002;**51**:324–5.
8. Centers for Disease Control and Prevention. Malaria Surveillance – United States, 2005. *MMWR.* 2007;**56**(SS06):23–38.
9. Centers for Disease Control and Prevention. Update: outbreak of acute febrile illness among athletes participating in Eco-Challenge-Sabah 2000—Borneo, Malaysia, 2000. *MMWR* 2001;**50**:21–4.
10. Connor BA. Sequelae of traveler's diarrhea: focus on postinfectious irritable bowel syndrome. *Clin Infect Dis* 2005;**1**(41 Suppl 8):S577–86.
11. Cunha BA. The clinical significance of fever patterns. *Infect Dis Clin North Am* 1996;**10**:33–42.
12. Doherty JF, Grant AD, Bryceson AD. Fever as the presenting complaint of travellers returning from the tropics. *QJM* 1995;**88**:277–81.
13. Franco-Paredes C. The Post-travel period. In: Arguin P, Kozarky P, Reed C, editors. *CDC Health Information for International Travel 2008. Centers for Disease Control and Prevention.* Mosby: Elsevier; 2007.
14. Freedman DO, Leder K. Influenza: changing approaches to prevention and treatment in travelers. *J Travel Med* 2005;**12**:36–44.
15. Hill DR. Health problems in a large cohort of Americans traveling to developing countries. *J Travel Med* 2000;**7**(5):259–66.
16. Hill DR. The burden of illnesses in international travelers. *N Engl J Med* 2007;**352**:115–7.
17. Jelinek T, Muhlberger N, Harms G, Grobusch MP, Knobloch J, Bronner U, et al. Epidemiology and clinical features of imported dengue fever in Europe: sentinel surveillance data from TropNetEurope. *Clin Infect Dis* 2002;**35**(9):1047–52.
18. Jensenius M, Fournier PE, Raoult D. Rickettsiosis in international travelers. *Clin Infect Dis* 2004;**39**:1493–9.

19. Jensenius M, Davis X, von Sonnenburg F, Schwartz E, Keystone JS, Leder K, Lopéz-Véléz R, Caumes E, Cramer JP, Chen L, and Parola P, for the GeoSentinel Surveillance Network Multicenter GeoSentinel Analysis of Rickettsial Diseases in International Travelers, 1996–2008. *Emerg Infect Dis* 2009;**15**,:1791–1798.

20. Matteelli A, Carosi G. Sexually transmitted diseases in travelers. *Clin Infect Dis* 2001;**32**:1063–7.

21. Mutsch M, Spicher VM, Gut C, Steffen R. Hepatitis A virus infections in travelers, 1988–2004. *Clin Infect Dis* 2006;**42**:490–7.

22. Newman RD, Parise ME, Barber AM, Steketee RW. Malaria-related deaths among U.S. travelers, 1963–2001. *Ann Intern Med* 2004;**141**:547–55.

23. O'Brien D, Tobin S, Brown GB, Torresi J. Fever in returned travelers: review of hospital admissions for a 3-year period. *Clin Infect Dis* 2001;**33**:603–9.

24. Ryan ET, Wilson ME, Kain KC. Illness after international travel. *N Engl J Med* 2002;**347**:505–16.

25. Schwartz E, Parise M, Kozarsky P, Cetron M. Delayed onset of malaria—implications for chemoprophylaxis in travelers. *N Engl J Med* 2003;**349**:1510–6.

26. Wilson ME, Weld LH, Boggild A, Keystone JS, Kain KC, van Sonnenburg F, et al. Fever in returned travelers results from the GeoSentinel surveillance network. *Clin Infect Dis* 2007;**44**:1560–8.

27. Wilson ME, Chen LH. Dermatologic infectious diseases in international travelers. *Curr Infect Dis Rep* 2004;**6**:54–62.

28. Hochberg N, Franco-Paredes C. Emerging infections in mobile populations. In: Scheld WM, Grayson ML, Hughes JM, editors. *Emerging Infections*. 9th ed. American Society of Microbiology Press; 2010.

Chapter 15

Infectious Syndromes Associated With Immunodeficiencies

DIAGNOSTIC APPROACH TO SELECTED PRIMARY AND SECONDARY IMMUNODEFICIENCIES

According to the 2015 phenotypic classification of primary immunodeficiencies, there are at this point approximately 300 single-gene inborn errors of immunity with phenotypes as diverse as leading to susceptibility to infection (eg, occurrence of severe influenza sepsis), allergy, autoimmunity (eg, systemic lupus erythematosus), autoinflammation (eg, Crohn's disease), and to the occurrence of malignancies.[1] Categories contained in the current classification of primary immunodeficiencies[1] are depicted in Table 15.1. Clinical syndromes associated with splenectomy or functional asplenia are discussed in chapter: Cutaneous, Subcutaneous, and Deep-Tissue Infections and chapter: Febrile Syndromes.

COMBINED VARIABLE IMMUNODEFICIENCY

Common variable immunodeficiency (CVID), if not severe and life threatening immediately in early infancy or childhood, is usually not diagnosed until 10–20 years after the onset of clinical signs and symptoms of the specific immunodeficiency.[2,3] Core concepts regarding the underlying defects and associated clinical syndromes with CVID are noted in Table 15.2. CVID is a primary immunodeficiency disorder characterized by hypogammaglobulinemia and a spectrum of other associated phenotypes. CVID is one of the most frequent immunodeficiency identified in humans. The underlying humoral deficiency in CVID is a quantitative deficiency of IgG usually accompanied by reduced levels of IgA and IgM.

OTHER IMMUNODEFICIENCIES CAUSED BY ANTIBODY DEFICIENCIES

Antibody deficiency may be present in the context of an inherited genetic defect associated with a specific primary immune deficiency; or as part of a range of secondary conditions (acquired). The main causes of secondary antibody deficiency are B-cell lymphoproliferative disorders (ie, chronic lymphocytic leukemia and multiple myeloma), protein-losing states such as nephrotic

Core Concepts in Clinical Infectious Diseases (CCCID). http://dx.doi.org/10.1016/B978-0-12-804423-0.00015-9
187

TABLE 15.1 Phenotypic Classification for Primary Immunodeficiencies[a]

Category	Phenotype (example)
Immunodeficiencies affecting cellular and humoral immunity	Severe combined immunodeficiency (SCID)
Combined immunodeficiency with associated or syndromic features	Hyper-IgE syndromes (HIES)
Predominantly antibody deficiencies with recurrent bacterial infections including otitis, pneumonia, sinusitis, diarrhea, sepsis	Common variable immunodeficiency disorders (CVID)
Diseases of immune dysregulation	Hemophagocytic lymphohistiocytosis
Congenital defects of phagocyte number, function, or both	Chronic granulomatous disease (CGD)
Defects in intrinsic and innate immunity	Chronic mucocutaneous candidiasis (CMC)
Autoinflammatory disorders	Familial mediterranean fever (FMF)
Complement deficiencies	*Neisseria* infections due to terminal complex deficiencies
Phenocopies of primary immunodeficiencies	Syndromes caused by autoantibodies to cytokines

[a]*Bousfiha A, Jeddane L, Al-Herz W, Ailal F, Casanova JL, Chatila T, et al. The 2015 IUIS phenotyphic classification for primary immunodeficiencies.* J Clin Immunol 2015;**35**(8):727–738 .

syndrome or protein-losing enteropathy, disorders of lymphatic circulation, and increased catabolism of immunoglobulins (Table 15.2). Additionally, currently available immune mediated therapies (monoclonal antibodies to other B-cell-targeted interventions) are responsible for many iatrogenic causes of antibody deficiency states.

The function of B-lymphocytes should be performed by quantitatively measuring antibody levels, determination of vaccination responses to selected antigens, and frequency of infections. At-risk patients should be followed closely, particularly if presenting with an infectious process that may rapidly evolve into severe sepsis or septic shock and thus immunoglobulin replacement therapy may offer a better clinical outcome along with antimicrobial and supportive therapy.[2–4]

IMMUNODEFICIENCIES ASSOCIATED WITH AUTOANTIBODIES TO CYTOKINES

There is an increasing recognition of phenocopies of primary immunodeficiency disorders characterized by the presence of autoantibodies targeting essential proteins of the canonical cytokine response resulting in a predisposition to specific clinical syndromes of infectious diseases or specific infectious pathogens[1,4–7] (Table 15.3).

TABLE 15.2 Etiology and Differential Diagnosis of Immunodeficiencies Associated with Antibody Deficiencies

Category	Etiology	Core concepts
Common variable immunodeficiency (CVID)[a]	Failure of B-cell differentiation and antibody secretion associated with other abnormalities in other components of the immune system leading to different clinical phenotypes	*Associated infections* Sinopulmonary infections Gastrointestinal infections (*Giardia lamblia, Campylobacter jejuni*) *Salmonella* spp. infections *Mycoplasma* spp. septic arthritis Enteroviral meningoencephalitis *Bronchiectasis and chronic respiratory tract infections* *Interstitial lung disease, granulomata, and lymphoproliferation* Granulomatous lymphocytic interstitial lung disease (GLILD), lymphocytic interstitial pneumonitis, lymphoid hyperplasia, and follicular bronchitis *Gastrointestinal complications* *H. pylori* associated diseases (gastric carcinoma and MALToma) CVID enteropathy with malabsorption and CVID large bowel (colitis) *Autoimmunity* Autoimmune cytopenias (ITP, hemolytic anemias) Rheumatoid arthritis Systemic lupus erythematosus Sicca syndrome Pernicious anemia *Malignancy* Gastric carcinoma Non-Hodgkin's lymphoma Other: breast carcinomas, ovarian carcinoma, multiple myeloma
Secondary hypogammaglobulinemia	Hematologic disorders Acquired disorders	Chronic lymphocytic leukemia Multiple myeloma Waldenström macroglobulinemia Lymphoma Primary amyloidosis Drug induced Transplantation Primary chylous disorders Splenectomy Chronic intestinal pseudoobstruction Protein-losing enteropathy Intestinal lymphangiectasia Nephrotic syndrome

TABLE 15.2 Etiology and Differential Diagnosis of Immunodeficiencies Associated with Antibody Deficiencies (*cont.*)

Category	Etiology	Core concepts
Primary combined immunodeficiency states associated with hypogamma-globulinemia[b]	X-linked	X-linked severe combined immunodeficiency (IL-2 receptor common γ chain Wiskott–Aldrich syndrome, X-linked thrombocytopenia Agammaglobulinemia and growth hormone (GH) deficiency, and others
	Autosomal	JAK3 deficiency (JAK 3) ADA deficiency (adenosine deaminase deficiency) DiGeorge syndrome (TBX1) Ataxia-Telangiectasia (ATM) Chronic mucocutaneous candidiasis (AIRE)[c]
Drug-induced antibody deficiencies	Rituximab	Anti-CD20 monoclonal antibody when used for autoimmune diseases (IgG4-related disease, eosinophilic granulmomatosis and polyangiitis, and others)
	CD 19-targeted chimeric antigen receptor T cells	CART used for acute lymphoblastic leukemia
	Atacicept	Used in multiple sclerosis and lupus-induced nephritis
	Imatinib	Used in chronic myelogenous leukemia
	Mycophenolate mofetil	Transplantation-induced immunosuppression
	Antiepileptic drugs	Carbamazepine, valproate, and phenytoin
	Cyclophosphamide	Used in systemic vasculitis, lupus nephritis
	Corticosteroids	Used in doses to modulate systemic inflammatory diseases including vasculitis or inflammatory disorders
	Sulfazalaine	Used in the treatment of inflammatory bowel disease
	Penicillamine	Used in Wilson's disease, rheumatoid arthritis

[a]Weiler CR, Bankers-Fulbright J. Common variable immunodeficiency: test indications and interpretations. Mayo Clin Proc 2005;**80**(9):1187–1200.
[b]There are many other X-linked and autosomal combined immunodeficiency states matched to specific genetic defects (Bousfiha A, Jeddane L, Al-Herz W, Ailal F, Casanova JL, Chatila T, et al. The 2015 IUIS Phenotypic classification for primary immunodeficiencies. J Clin Immunol 2015;35(8):727–738.
[c]Yong PFK, Tarzi M, Chua I, Grimbacher B, Chee R. Common variable immunodeficiency: an update on etiology and management. Immunol Allergy Clin N Am 2008;**28**:367–386.

TABLE 15.3 Clinical Spectrum of Immunodeficiencies Associated with Anticytokine Antibodies

Category of autoantibodies[a]	Diseases/syndromes
Autoantibodies to Factor H of the Complement cascade (Antifactor H autoantibodies)	Atypical hemolytic uremic syndrome (trombothic microangiophathy)
Autoantibodies to interleukin-17 (IL-17) and/or interleukin 22 (IL-22) (Anti-IL-17 autoantibodies, anti-IL-22 autoantibodies)	Chronic mucocutaneous candidiasis (CMC)
Autoantibodies to interleukin-6 (IL-6) (anti-IL-6 autoantibodies)	Recurrent skin infections
Autoantibodies to interferon-gamma (IFN-γ) (anti-IFN- γ autoantibodies)	Mendelian susceptibility to mycobacteria disease (MSMD) or combined immunodeficiency (CID) Mycobacterial, fungal, *Salmonella*, Varicella–Zoster virus infections
Autoantibodies to C1 inhibitor (C_1 esterase) (anti-C_1 INH)	Angioedema
Autoantibodies to granulocyte macrophage colony stimulating factor (GM-CSF) (anti-GM-CSF autoantibodies)	Pulmonary alveolar proteinosis Meningoencephalitis caused by *Cryptococcus gattii*

[a]*Bousfiha A, Jeddane L, Al-Herz W, Ailal F, Casanova JL, Chatila T, et al. The 2015 IUIS Phenotypic classification for primary immunodeficiencies. J Clin Immunol 2015;35(8):727–738.*

CHRONIC GRANULOMATOUS DISEASE

Chronic granulomatous disease (CGD) is caused by an impaired oxygen metabolism in phagocytes and the resultant of mutations in any of the five structural genes of the NADPH oxidase enzyme.[8] NADPH oxidase catalyzes the transfer of an electrom from cytoplasmic NADPH to molecular oxygen. Defects in the function of this enzyme lead to phagocyte dysfunction caused by a faulty oxidative burst phenomenon. Mutations in all of the five structural genes of NADPH oxidase can cause CGD. Mutations in the gp 91^{phox} gen accounts for approximately 65% of cases of CGD. The most frequent clinical syndromes associated to an increased predisposition to infection include skin, lung, lymph nodes, and liver syndromes. The majority of infections in CGD in North America include pathogens such as *Staphylococcus aureus, Serratia marcescens, Burkholderia cepacia* complex (ie, *Burkholderia gladioli*), *Chromobacterium violaceum, Francisella philomiragia, Granulibacter bethesdensis, Nocardia* spp., and *Aspergillus* spp. (ie, *Aspergillus nidulans*) and other fungal pathogens (*Paecilomyces variotti, Paecilomyces lilacinus, and Neosartorya udagawae*). Fungal elements may elicit an exuberant inflammatory response in CGD such as it may occur with Mulch pneumonitis (when an individual with CGD is exposed to decaying organic matter). In addition, patients with CGD may develop severe localized infection caused by BCG vaccination (Bacille–Calmette–Guérin). There is also inflammatory-related diseases in CGD including a Crohn's-like disease, or nonspecific inflammation throughout the gastrointestinal tract; discoid lupus erythematosus-like lesions, aphtous ulcers and photosensitivity among those who are carriers of gp 91^{phox}.

The era of antibiotic prophylaxis among immunocompromised hosts began with CGD. The use of trimethoprim-sulfamethoxazole substantially reduced the frequency of bacterial infections in this population. More recently, the institution of azole prophylaxis to prevent *Aspergillus* spp. infections has led to a reduced mortality rate in CGD. The use of glucocorticoids along with antimicrobials also has been shown to be clinically useful in cases of liver abscesses. Currently, bone-marrow transplantation can lead to remission of CGD.[9]

COMPLEMENT DEFICIENCIES

A key component of the innate immune response is the group of related-proteins designated as the complement system[9] (Table 15.4). Activation of the complement through different pathways (classic, alternative, and lectin) is considered as a central event in combating infections and in the regulation of the innate and acquired immune responses. Deficiencies of selective components of the complement system can be associated with an increased susceptibility to pathogens or to a predisposition to develop autoimmune or autoinflammatory diseases.[1] Predisposition to neisserial infections is usually determined by defects leading to the inappropriate construction of the membrane attack complex (MAC), which is formed by the sequential fusion of C6, C7, C8, and C9–C5b. The formation of MAC confers its ability to bind to the membrane of microorganisms to form a transmembrane pore that disrupts the intracellular milieu of these organisms favoring their death.

NEUTROPENIA

This is a common form of secondary immunosuppression and the direct result of potent immunosuppressive chemotherapeutic agents in the treatment of cancer.[6] The perfect storm in this syndrome is achieved with two pathogenic events: (1) reduced number and function of polymorphonuclear cells as a result of direct toxicity of myeloid precursors in the bone marrow; and (2) bystander injury to rapidly dividing cells particularly epithelial cells. Thus, there is rapid mucosal affection of the gastrointestinal mucosal lining leading to the translocation of potentially pathogen microorganisms. By simply having marrow injury caused by HIV-infection or drug-induced myelosupression, patients with HIV/AIDS presenting with neutropenia, do not represent a clinically severe and potentially life threatening situation compared with some undergoing chemotherapy for acute myelogenous leukemia developing neutropenia, where mucosal damage is present as a risk factor for bacteremia and sepsis[10] (Table 15.5).

TABLE 15.4 Complement Deficiencies and Infectious Diseases[a]

Category[b]	Etiology	Core concepts
High susceptibility to infections	Recurrent pyogenic infections	Deficiency of C3 LOF (C3 loss of function) Deficiency of MASP2 (mannan-binding lectin –MBL-associated serine protease 2) Deficiency of Ficolin 3 (FCN3) manifesting as recurrent severe pyogenic infections mainly in the lungs; selective antibody defect to pneumococcal polysaccharides, and necrotizing enterocolitis in infancy
	Neisserial infections	Deficiency of CR3 (ITGAM) Deficiency of Factor H (CFH) associated with membranoproliferative glomerulonephritis *Neisserial infections only* Deficiency of properdin (PFC) Deficiency of C9 Deficiency of factor D (CFD) *Neisserial infections and systemic lupus Erythematosus* Deficiency of C6 Deficiency of C8A Deficiency of C8G Deficiency of C5 *Neisserial infections and vasculitis* Deficiency of C7
Low susceptibility to infections	SLE-like syndrome	Rheumatoid disease and infections Deficiency of C4 (C4A, C4B) Deficiency of C1q (C1QA, C1QB, C1QC) Deficiency of C1R Infections, vasculitis and polymyositis Deficiency of C2 Infections and multiple autoimmune diseases
	Atypical hemolytic uremic syndrome	Deficiency of C1s (C1S) Deficiency of membrane cofactor protein (CD46) associated with glomerulonephritis and of autosomal dominant inheritance pattern Deficiency of Factor B, Factor H-related (CFHR1-5)
	Others	Deficiency of thrombomodulin (THBD) Deficiency of C3GOF (C3 gain of function) Deficiency of C1 inhibitor (SERPING 1) associated with hereditary angioedema and of autosomal dominant inheritance pattern Deficiency of CD59 (MIRL) associated with hemolytic anemia and thrombosis

[a]*Ram S, Lewis LA, Rice PA. Infections of people with complement deficiencies and patients who have undergone splenectomy. Clin Microb Rev 2010;23(4):740–780.*
[b]*Bousfiha A, Jeddane L, Al-Herz W, Ailal F, Casanova JL, Chatila T, et al. The 2015 IUIS Phenotypic classification for primary immunodeficiencies. J Clin Immunol 2015;35(8):727–738.*

TABLE 15.5 Clinical Spectrum of Selected Neutropenic Febrile Syndromes[a]

Category	Etiology	Core concepts
Fungal pathogens	Invasive candidiasis (*Candida albicans, C. tropicalis* in Bone Marrow Transplantation -)	Hepatosplenic candidiasis Candidemia Myositis
	Fusariosis (*Fusarium* spp.)	Multiple skin lesions (multiple erythematous macules with central pallor that quickly evolve into papules and necrotic nodules in the extremities but may occur in the trunk and face)
	Cryptococcus spp.	May manifest as cryptococcemia, meningoencephalitis, soft and tissue infections (cellulitis), and pneumonia
	Trichosporon beigelii	Disseminated fungal infection with skin lesions (macules to maculopapular lesions), can be confused with *Candida* spp.
	Aspergillus spp.	Aspergillus fumigatus is the most commonly isolated species in neutropenic patients followed by *A. flavus, A. niger,* and *A. terreus* usually manifesting as invasive pulmonary aspergillosis or disseminated aspergillosis with central nervous involvement
	Rhizopus and *Mucor* spp.	Confluent areas of necrosis to a necrotizing vascular infiltration, may occur in the skin or in the head and neck, or pulmonary (seen when voriconazole is used as prophylaxis among transplanted patients)
	Reactivation of endemic dimorphic fungi	*Histoplasma capsulatum* *Coccidiodes immitis* *Blastomyces dermatitides*
Bacterial pathogens	Gram-negative bacilli	Pseudomonas aeruginosa Klebsiella pneumonia (KPC-producer) *E. coli* ESBL producer
	Gram-positive cocci	Viridans group Streptococci *S. aureus* (MRSA or MSSA) Vancomycin Resistant Enterococci Group A, B, C, E Streptococci *Leuconostoc* spp. Invasive *Streptococcus pneumoniae*
	Gram-positive rods	*Lactobacillus* spp. *Corynebacterium jeikeium* *Bacillus* spp. Listeria monocytogenenes *Propionibacterium acnes*

TABLE 15.5 Clinical Spectrum of Selected Neutropenic Febrile Syndromes (*cont.*)

Category	Etiology	Core concepts
Viral pathogens	Severe influenza Respiratory syncytial virus	Rapidly progressive Respiratory failure and sepsis
Specific clinical syndromes	Hepatosplenic candidiasis	Among patients recovering from neutropenia, manifesting as persistent episodes of fever, elevation of alkaline phosphatase level
	Neutropenic enterocolitis (often associated with *Clostridium septicum*)	Typhlitis
	Necrotizing gingivitis Catheter-associated Bloodstream Infections	Mixed oral flora including anaerobes Bloodstream infections and tunnel catheters (sometimes unusual organisms such as *Mycobacterium fortuitum*, *Corynebacterium jeikeum* may be isolated)
	Invasive pulmonary Aspergillosis Rhinocerebral Mucormycosis	
Miscellaneous conditions mimicking infectious process[a]	Neutrophilic dermatoses Pulmonary infiltrates and Fever[b]	Sweet's syndrome Idiopathic pneumonia syndrome in posthematopoietic stem cell transplantation

ESBL, Extended spectrum beta-lactamase; KPC, Klebsiella pneumoniae carbapenemase producer.
[a]*Intracellular pathogens have been associated with T-cell deficiencies resulting in increased risk of* Listeria monocytogenes, Salmonella spp, Mycobacterium tuberculosis, Cryptococcus neoformans. *Among patients with central nervous malignancies and those with acute lymphocytic leukemia, receiving extremely high doses of glucocorticoids are a substantially increased risk of cryptococcosis and* Pneumocystis jiroveci *pneumonia (PCP), and disseminated strongyloidiasis.*
[b]*This is an acute lung dysfunction of non-infectious etiology and considered a complication following hematopoietic stem cell transplantation wit widespread alveolar injury, absence of infection, and no cardiac or renal etiology (Panoskaltsis-Mortar A, Griese M, Madtes DK, Belperio JA, Hadda IY, Folz RJ. Am J Respir Crit Care Med 2011;183:1262–1279).*

IMMUNODEFICIENCY ASSOCIATED WITH HIV/AIDS

HIV/AIDS can be associated with a broad range of clinical syndromes including fever and neurologic syndrome, pulmonary syndromes, gastrointestinal syndromes, dermatologic syndromes, genitourinary syndromes, and others (Table 15.6).

TABLE 15.6 Selected Clinical Syndromes Among Patients with HIV/AIDS

Category	Etiology
Fever and pulmonary infiltrates	Community-acquired pneumonia *Pneumocystis jiroveci* pneumonia (PCP) Drug-induced hypersensitivity Active pulmonary tuberculosis Coccidiodomycosis *Penicillium marneffei* Kaposi's sarcoma
Fever and lymphadenopathy	Disseminated tuberculosis Disseminated histoplasmosis Lymphoma Bacillary angiomatosis (*Bartonella henselae*) Castleman's disease (HHV-8 Associated)[a]
Fever with/without severe and persistent diarrhea	*Cryptosporidium* spp. *Isospora belli* Nontyphoidal Salmonellosis CMV colitis *Campylobacter* spp. *Shigella flexneri* or *Shigella Sonnei* *Clostridium difficile* colitis *Mycobacterium avium-intracellulare*
Cholangitis	*Cryptosporidium* *Mycobacterium-avium intracellulare* CMV colangiopathy
Neurologic syndromes	*Toxoplasma gondii* (toxoplasma encephalitis, chorioretinitis) JC virus (polyoma) Cryptococcal meningoenchepalitis Primary central nervous system lymphona (Epstein–Barr associated) CMV encephalopathy, polyradiculopathy, retinitis VZV associated diseases (encephalitis, meningitis, acute retinal necrosis)
Pancytopenia, fever, and elevated liver enzymes	Disseminated histoplasmosis Hemophagocytic syndrome ADAMTS-13 thrombotic microangiopathy lymphoma (Epstein–Barr associated, ie, Burkitt's lymphoma) Human granulocytic ehrlichiosis Visceral leishmaniasis (*Leishmania donovani/Leishmania infantum* complex)
Immune reconstitution syndromes	Tuberculosis Cryptococcosis-related Hepatitis B-related Kaposi's sarcoma (HHV-8) associated (KRAS)

TABLE 15.6 Selected Clinical Syndromes Among Patients with HIV/AIDS (*cont.*)

Category	Etiology
Dermatologic	Syphilis (primary or secondary including malignant lues) Umbilicated lesions (histoplasmosis, penicillinosis, or disseminated cryptococossis) Eosinophilic folliculitis HPV-related warts and carcinomas Molluscum contagiousum (pox virus)

[a]*HHV-8, Human herpes virus-8 (associated diseases include in coinfected patients with HIV: Kaposi's sarcoma, Castleman's disease, body cavity lymphoma, and possibly pulmonary hypertension).*

TABLE 15.7 Clinical Spectrum and Differential Diagnosis of Infections after Solid-Organ or Hematopoietic Transplantation

Temporal pattern[a]	Etiology[b]
First 30 days from transplantation	Colitis (*Clostridium difficile*) Urinary tract infections (MDR-Gram negative bacilli hospital acquired (ESBL-*E. coli* or *Klebsiella* spp.) Abdominal infections (polymicrobial, anaerobic gram-negative bacilli, enterococci, *Pseudomonas spp.*, MDR-gram negative bacilli hospital acquired (ESBL-*E. coli* or *Klebsiella* spp.) Herpes simplex, Varicella–Zoster virus reactivation syndromes Pneumonia (hospital-acquired *S. aureus* or Gram-negative bacilli –MDR) Candidemia or Staphylococci bloodstream infections
Day 31 to 6 months from transplantation	Infections caused by *Nocardia* spp, Tuberculosis (extrapulmonary), *Clostridium difficile*, *S. aureus*, Multidrug resistant gram-negative bacilli (hospital acquired) Candidiasis, Aspergillosis, Cryptococcus neoformans skin and soft tissue, pneumonia, cryptococcemia, meningoencephalitis Rhinocerebral mucor/rhizopus Reactivation of endemic dimorphic fungi Pneumocystis jiroveci pneumonia (PCP) Pulmonary toxoplasmosis (parasitic)
Beyond 6 months from transplantation	Invasive pneumococcal disease RSV, influenza Community acquired bacteria *Clostridium difficile* colitis Potential occurrence of infections mentioned during Day 31 to 6 months

MDR, Multidrug resistant
[a]*The risk for infections is determined by exposure history and degree of immunosuppression and by the medical history of the donor. The occurrence of some infectious processes may not follow a precise temporality, particularly due to the growing use of prophylactic antifungal, antibacterial, and sometime antiviral prophylactic regimens*
[b]*Fishman JA. Infection in solid-organ transplant recipients. N Engl J Med 2007;**357**(25):2601–2613.*

198 Core Concepts in Clinical Infectious Diseases (CCCID)

TABLE 15.8 Clinical Spectrum of Disease Associated with Infections in Patients with Diabetes Mellitus[a]

Condition	Core concepts
Group B Streptococci bacteremia	Strong association with diabetes mellitus
Klebsiella pneumoniae invasive syndrome	Liver abscess, endophtalmitis and liver abscess (abscesses) and bacteremia
Rhinocerebral mucormycosis (*Rhizopus* and *Mucor*)	During uncontrolled hyperglicemia and diabetic ketoacidosis
S. aureus bacteremia, cutaneous skin and soft tissue infections, and other related syndromes	Usually healthcare acquired strains but it may also be associated with community-acquired MRSA or MSSA strains
Salmonella enteritidis	In some studies reported to be highly associated with bacteremia in diabetic individuals
Malignant otitis externa	Associated with otomastoiditis caused by either *Pseudomonas aeruginosa* or *S. aureus*
Emphysematous pyelonephritis, papillary necrosis	*E. coli* is the most frequently identified facultative anaerobic pathogen
Emphysematous cholecystitis,	Presence of gallstones is a risk factor in a patient with diabetes mellitus.

[a]*Joshi N, Caputo GM, Weitekamp MR, Karchmer AW. Infections in patients with diabetes mellitus. N Engl J Med 1999;**341**(25):1906–1911.*

INFECTIONS ASSOCIATED WITH SOLID ORGAN AND HEMATOPOIETIC STEM CELL TRANSPLANTATION

The majority of infectious syndromes associated with transplantation are elicited by bacterial opportunistic pathogens, followed by fungi and viruses[11] (Table 15.7).

INFECTIONS ASSOCIATED WITH DIABETES MELLITUS

Persons with diabetes mellitus are at increased risk of suffering a plethora of clinical syndromes caused predominantly by bacterial and fungal pathogens[12] (Table 15.8).

REFERENCES

1. Bousfiha A, Jeddane L, Al-Herz W, Ailal F, Casanova JL, Chatila T, et al. The 2015 IUIS Phenotypic classification for primary immunodeficiencies. *J Clin Immunol* 2015; doi: 10.1007/s10875-015-0198-5.
2. Weiler CR, Bankers-Fulbright J. Common variable immunodeficiency: test indications and interpretations. *Mayo Clin Proc* 2005;**80**(9):1187–200.
3. Yong PFK, Tarzi M, Chua I, Grimbacher B, Chee R. Common variable immunodeficiency: an update on etiology and management. *Immunol Allergy Clin N Am* 2008;**28**:367–86.
4. Dhalla F, Misbah SA. Secondary antibody deficiencies. *Curr Opin Allergy Clin Immunol* 2015;**15**:503–13.
5. Saijo T, Chen J, Chen SCA, Rosen LB, Jin Y, Sorrell TC, et al. Anti-granulocyte macrophage colony-stimulating factor autoantibodies are a risk factor for central nervous infection by *Cryptococcus gattii* in otherwise immunocompetent patients. *mBio* 2014;**5**(2):1–8.
6. Patel SM, Sekiguchi H, Reynolds JP, Krowka MJ. Pulmonary alveolar proteinosis. *Can Resp J* 2012;**19**(4):243–53.
7. Browne SK, Burbelo PD, Chetchotisakd P, Suputtamongkol Y, Kiertiburanakul S, Shaw P, et al. Adult-onset immunodeficiency in Thailand and Taiwan. *N Engl J Med* 2012;**367**(8):725–34.
8. Holland SM. Chronic granulomatous disease. *Hematol Oncol Clin North Am* 2013;**27**(1):89–99.
9. Ram S, Lewis LA, Rice PA. Infections of people with complement deficiencies and patients who have undergone splenectomy. *Clin Microb Rev* 2010;**23**(4):740–80.
10. Alp S, Akova M. Management of febrile neutropenia in the era of bacterial resistance. *Ther Adv Infect Dis* 2013;**1**(1):37–43.
11. Fishman JA. Infection in solid-organ transplant recipients. *N Engl J Med* 2007;**357**(25):2601–13.
12. Joshi N, Caputo GM, Weitekamp MR, Karchmer AW. Infections in patients with diabetes mellitus. *N Engl J Med* 1999;**341**(25):1906–11.

Chapter 16

Specific Organ Syndromes

RHABDOMYOLYSIS

This syndrome is characterized by muscle necrosis with the spillage of intramuscular contents into the bloodstream leading to myoglobinuria, which in turn can may lead acute kidney injury. There are three main mechanisms of damage: (1) nontraumatic exertional damage to the muscle; (2) nontraumatic and nonexertional (drugs, toxins, or infections); and (3) traumatic muscle compression (prolonged immobilization and crush injury). The most frequent causes of rhabdomyolysis in clinical practice include influenza A and B, and community-acquired pneumonia caused by Legionella pneumophila. However, there are many other microorganisms that could potentially cause rhabdomyolysis (Table 16.1).

ACID–BASE DISORDERS AND INFECTIOUS DISEASES

There are two main types of acid–base disturbances, metabolic and respiratory.[1] Identifying the acid–base status of a patient assists you in terms of diagnosis and also provides the opportunity to follow these parameters to assess response to therapy. Some core concepts about acid–base disorders in the setting of an infectious disease include the following:

- Infection diseases may be associated with specific acid–base disturbances.
- Food poisoning may be associated with a chloride responsive metabolic alkalosis given the pronounced vomiting associated with for some conditions (eg, *Bacillus cereus* producing emetic toxin).
- Similarly, respiratory alkalosis and in fact, it is considered as a criteria of the systemic inflammatory response (SIRS – respiratory rate >20 or a $PaCO_2$ <25 mmHg) and it is often seen during an episode of acute respiratory failure; sometimes associated with acute lung injury caused by Gram-negative bacilli sepsis.
- Mixed acid–base disorders may also occur when a metabolic acidosis caused by lactic acidosis due to tissue hypoperfusion is present in an individual with severe sepsis or septic shock and with associated respiratory alkalosis as part of SIRS.
- Patients with acute respiratory acidosis due to hypoventilation are prone to large volume aspiration and therefore may develop aspiration pneumonitis.

Core Concepts in Clinical Infectious Diseases (CCCID). http://dx.doi.org/10.1016/B978-0-12-804423-0.00016-0

TABLE 16.1 Infectious Causes of Rhabdomyolysis[a,b]

Category	Description	Core concepts
Viral	Influenza A and B Parainfluenza virus HIV Epstein–Barr virus (EBV) Herpes simplex virus Varicella Zoster virus (VZV) Echovirus Cytomegalovirus Adenovirus	Sometimes creatinine-phosphokinase levels may be higher than 100,000 in patients with sepsis due to influenza A
Legionnaire's disease	Community acquired pneumonia	Frequent cause of rhabdomyolysis associated with hypophosphatemia, elevated liver enzymes and sometimes hyponatremia
Other Bacterial	Bacterial pyomyositis *Francisella tularensis* *Coxiella burnetti* *S. aureus* bacteremia/sepsis *S. pyogenes*	
Rickettsial	Human granulocytic ehrlichiosis (*E. chaffeensis*)	More frequently than other rickettsial diseases including Rocky Mountain spotted fever
Drug induced	Daptomycin[c] Trimethoprim/sulfamethoxazole Macrolides (clarithromycin)	Used in the treatment of *S. aureus* bacteremia
Toxin mediated	*S. aureus* *S. pyogenes*	Toxic shock syndrome Toxic shock syndrome

[a]*Allison RC, Bedsole L. The other medical causes of Rhabdomyolysis. Am J Med Sci 2003;326(2):79–88.*
[b]*Singh U, Scheld WM. Infectious etiologies of Rhabdomyolysis: three cases reports and review. Clin Infect Dis 1996;22:642–649.*
[c]*In some instances, when CPK is increasing, it is reasonable to stop a statin drug used in the long-term treatment of hyperlipidemia during treatment with daptomycin. Occasionally, daptomycin may also be associated with an eosinophilic pneumonia manifesting soon after its initiation.*

Depending on the volume and contents of gastric material, as well as on the amount and types of oral commensal bacteria (viridans group streptococci, Gram-positive anaerobic oral commensals, and others), a bacterial pneumonitis, lung abscess, and/or empyema may develop.

- Large amounts of transfused packed-red blood cells during shock, trauma, or among surgical patients may cause a transfusion-induced alkalosis.
- Diarrhea secondary to enterophathogens such as enterotoxigenic *Escherichia coli* or *Vibrio cholera* may produce a severe hyperchloremic acidosis; or a mixed acidosis.

ELECTROLYTE ABNORMALITIES AND INFECTIOUS DISEASES

Electrolyte imbalances are often associated with critically ill patients in the medical ward or in the intensive care unit. Some electrolyte abnormalities may be exacerbated by an active infectious disease or as side effects of specific antimicrobial therapies (Table 16.2). Some of these electrolyte abnormalities add significant morbidity and mortality.

TABLE 16.2 Electrolyte Abnormalities and Infectious Diseases[a]

Electrolyte disturbance	Associated infections	Core concepts
Hyponatremia	*Hypertonic hyponatremia*	Infection induced hyperglycemia
	Isotonic hyponatremia (due to hyperproteinemia –hypergammaglobu-linemia)	HCV, HIV, and Visceral leishmaniasis
	Hypotonic hyponatremia	
	• Hypovolemic hyponatremia	Extrarenal Na^+ loss due to diarrhea or vomiting or adrenal insufficiency (renal loss of Na^+)
	• Euvolemic hyponatremia	Syndrome of inappropriate secretion of antidiuretic hormone (SIADH) due to increased production from lung parenchyma –active tuberculosis *Legionella pneumophila* Community-acquired pneumonia PCP

(Continued)

TABLE 16.2 Electrolyte Abnormalities and Infectious Diseases (*cont.*)

Electrolyte disturbance	Associated infections	Core concepts
	• Hypervolemic hyponatremia (edema)	*Nephrotic syndrome* (due to hepatitis B or HIV) *Cirrhosis of the liver* Chronic viral hepatitis B Chronic viral hepatitis C *Congestive heart failure* Coxsackie or echo induced cardiomyopathy due to acute myocarditis Dilated cardiomyopathy associated with Chagas disease (*Trypanosoma cruzi*) *Drug induced* High dose trimethoprim/ sulfamethoxazole during *Pneumocystis jiroveci* pneumonia (PCP) (intravenous formulations of trimethoprim/ sulfamethoxazole are usually mixed with D5W 5% glucose and 95% free water)
Hypernatremia	Diabetes insipidus	*S. pneumoniae* bacterial meningitis Tuberculous meningitis
Hyperkalemia	High-dose trimethoprim/ sulfamethoxazole during PCP Metabolic acidosis due to lactic acidosis secondary during tissue hypoperfusion of gram-negative sepsis	Caused by trimethoprim component
Hypokalemia	*P. falciparum* malaria *Cryptosporidium* diarrhea Enterocolitis syndromes	Associated with hyponatremia
	Drug induced	Amphotericin B formulations (also associated with hypomagnesemia and acute kidney injury)

TABLE 16.2 Electrolyte Abnormalities and Infectious Diseases (*cont.*)

Electrolyte disturbance	Associated infections	Core concepts
Hypercalcemia	HTLV-1	Adult T-cell leukemia/lymphoma Increased granulomatous response (chronic granulomatous processes)
	Mycobaterial	*M. tuberculosis*
	Fungal	Coccidiodomycosis and Histoplasmosis
	Bacterial	*Nocardia* infection of the lung/brain Brucellosis
Hypocalcemia	Staphylococci or streptococci induced toxic shock syndrome Sepsis due to gram-negative bacilli	It is postulated that it is due to increased production of procalcitonin and also due to hypoalbuminemia Associated with low ionized calcium (not as often in gram-positive sepsis)
Hypophosphatemia	Staphylococci toxic shock syndrome *Legionella pneumophila* community-acquired pneumonia	It may also be identified during severe sepsis caused both gram-positive and gram-negative bacteria

[a]*Liamis G, Milionis HJ, Elisaf M. Hyponatremia in patients with infectious diseases. J Infect 2011;**63**:327–335.*

ENDOCRINE ORGANS AND INFECTIOUS DISEASES

Pituitary Dysfunction

Pituitary abscesses may be secondary to bacterial meningitis (*Streptococcus pneumoniae*) or tuberculous meningitis. Fungal infections may spread to the pituitary gland in the case of histoplasmosis, blastomycosis, and coccidiodomycosis. Pituitary abscesses have been described with *Trypanosoma brucei rhodesiense* (sleeping sickness). Finally, viral infections such as poliomyelitis, influenza, mumps, measles, and St. Louis encephalitis have been associated with pituitary dysfunction. All of these infectious processes, and depending on the degree of involvement of the anterior and posterior pituitary gland, may manifest as either diabetes insipidus during the immediate process or may develop long-term sequelae manifested as either hypogonadism, central diabetes insipidus, hypothyroidism, central adrenal insufficiency, and/or growth abnormalities.[2]

Thyroid Disorders

There are two potential conditions that need to be discussed in this section. Acute suppurative thyroiditis and subacute thryoidtis which could be of viral origin. The former can be caused by fungal, mycobacterial, bacterial, or parasitic infections. Acute bacterial thyroiditis is more common in women and in those with preexisting thyroid disease and it may present with dysphagia, anterior neck pain and tenderness. Most common bacterial pathogens include *Staphylococus aureus, Streptococcus pyogenes, S. pneumoniae, Enterobacter spp, Salmonella, Yersinia enterocolitica, and Actinomyces.*

Gonads

Epididymo-orchitis is often acquired sexually in younger individuals and usually caused by *Chlamydia* and gonococci. In older adults, gram-negative bacilli are more frequently identified (*E. coli, Klebisella* spp). However, the two most relevant conditions to mention include mumps-associated orchitis, and erythema nodosum leprosum (type 2 leprosy reaction). Other viral infections associated with epididymo-orchitis include Epstein–Barr virus, echovirus 6, parvovirus B19, and Coxsackie B and A9. Hydrocele may also be associated with enlarged scrotum due to lymphatic filariasis caused by *Wuchereria bancrofti* or *Brugyia malayi. Tuberculous orchitis*, nontuberculous mycobacteria (*Mycobacterium fortuitum, Mycobacterium kansasii*) and brucella orchitis have been described.

ADRENAL GLANDS

The Waterhouse–Friderichsen syndrome (WFS) is associated with some infectious diseases leading to substantial morbidity by producing acute adrenal insufficiency associated with hemorrhage and dysfunction of the suprarenal glands, at a time when their response is crucial to address acute stress (Table 16.3). In response to acute stress, adrenal changes result in increased size of the cortex, loss of liquids from the outer cortical zones, transudates and inflammatory exudates into the cell columns, and multiple scattered areas of thrombosis. However, in some individuals, there may be superimposed extensive hemorrhages inside the cortex and occasionally extending into the medulla, leading to severe adrenal insufficiency manifesting as the WHF. In addition to the WHF syndrome, some infectious pathogens may cause adrenal insufficiency including HIV, disseminated *Mycobacterium avium-intracellulare* infection, *Plasmodium falciparum* severe malaria (end organ damage or >5% parasitemia), and herpes encephalitis.

TABLE 16.3 Infectious Causes of the Waterhouse–Friderichsen Syndrome[a]

Disease	Associated conditions
Waterhouse–Friderichsen syndrome	*Infectious*
	Meningococcemia (initial description of the syndrome) *S. aureus* bacteremia[b] Group A Streptococci (*S. pyogenes* invasive disease) Group B Streptococci (*S. agalactiae* invasive disease) *Pseudomonas aeruginosa* Invasive *S. pneumoniae* Disseminated *Histoplasma capsulatum* or *Histoplasma duboisii*
	Noninfectious
	Anticoagulation Antiphospholipid syndrome

[a]*Wheeler D, Amidon EL. Waterhouse–Friderichsen Syndrome. Report of a case with recovery.* N Engl J Med 1952;**247**(7):256–259.
[b]*Adem PV, Montgomery CP, Husain AN, Koogler TK, Arangelovich V, Humilier M, et al.* Staphylococcus aureus *sepsis and Waterhouse–Friderichsen syndrome in children.* N Engl J Med 2005;**353**(12)1245–1251.

In contrast to adrenal insufficiency, infectious diseases such as *Nocardia*, PCP, strongyloidiasis, and cryptococcosis can be associated with Cushing's syndrome due to excessive and prolonged production of glucocorticoids. A finding of calcification in the adrenal glands suggests previous history of tuberculosis, histoplasmosis, or adrenal hemorrhage.

Modulating the inflammatory response with glucocorticoids during infectious diseases has been studied in different clinical situations. The basis for addressing this question is the fact that in many instances the clinical manifestations and outcomes of some infectious disease processes directly depend from the host inflammatory response. In fact, despite effective sterilization of some infections with effective antimicrobial therapy, the morbidity and mortality of some infections has not improved. The main antiinflammatory modulation induced by steroids is the direct result of inhibiting the action of NF-Kβ activating genes associated with inflammatory cytokines IL-1, IL-2 and TNF-α (Table 16.4).

HEMATOLOGIC ABNORMALITIES

The syndrome of fever and pancytopenia is presented in detail in chapter: Febrile Syndromes. Fever and neutropenia, is discussed in chapter: Syndromes Associated With Immunodeficiencies. A diagnostic approach for fever and thrombocytopenia; and syndromes manifesting as fever and anemia is presented in Table 16.5.

TABLE 16.4 Efficacy of Corticosteroids in Improving Clinical Outcomes of Selected Infectious Diseases[a]

Disease category	Clinical impact
Tuberculous meningitis	Decreased neurologic sequelae and decreased mortality[b]
Tuberculous pericarditis	Decreased risk of fluid reaccumulation and thus reduced need for open pericardial window[c] but a recent trial neither prednisolone nor *M. indicus pranii* immunotherapy had a significant impact on death, cardiac tamponade requiring pericardiocentesis, or constrictive pericarditis[d]
Typhoid encephalopathy	Accelerates neurologic recovery among those with encephalopathy (delirium, stupor, or coma)[a]
Neurocysticercosis	Along with antiparasitic therapy decreased risk of partial seizures becoming[e] generalized
Streptococci cellulitis	Improves swelling and blistering[f]
Pneumocystic carinii pneumonia	Improves overall survival along with antimicrobial therapy (cotrimoxazole)[g]
Toxoplasma gondii encephalitis	Decreases cerebral edema surrounding lesions
Leprosy reactions	Type 1 (reversal reaction) Type 2 (erythema nodosum leprosum)[h]
Bacterial meningitis	Reduced mortality only when it was caused by *S. pneumoniae* in adults[i] Reduced neurologic sequelae in children with *Haemophilus influenzae*
Varicella–Zoster vasculopathy	Marked improvement in neurologic outcomes with steroids[j]
Chronic granulomatous disease (CGD)	Staphylococcal liver abscesses improve with the combination of antimicrobials and steroids without the need for surgical drainage

[a]McGowan JE, Chesney PJ, Crossley KB, LaForce FM. Guidelines for the use of systemic glucocorticosteroids in the management of selected infections. Clin Infect Dis 1992;**165**:1–13.
[b]Thwaites GE, Nguyen DB, Nguyen HD, Hoang TQ, Do TT, Nguyen TC, et al. Dexamethasone for the treatment of tuberculous meningitis in adolescents and adults. N Engl J Med 2004;**351**(17):1741–1751.
[c]Trautner BW, Darouiche RO. Tuberculous pericarditis: optimal diagnosis and management. Clin Infect Dis 2001;**33**(7): 954–961.
[d]Mayosi BM, Ntsekhe M, Bosch J, Pandie S, Jung H, Gumedze F, et al. Prednisolone and Mycobacterium indicus pranii in Tuberculous pericarditis. N Engl J Med 2015; **371**:1121–1130.
[e]Garcia HH, Pretell JE, Gilman RH, Martinez M, Moulton LH, Del Brutto O, et al. A trial of antiparasitic treatment to reduce seizures due to cerebral cysticercosis. N Engl J Med 2004;**350**:259–258.
[f]Stevens DL, Bisno AL, Chambers HF, Everett ED, Dellinger P, Goldstein EJC, et al. Practice guidelines for the diagnosis and management of skin and soft–tissue infections. Clin Infect Dis 2005;**41**:1373–1406.
[g]Bozzette SA, Sattler FR, Chiu J, Wu AW, Gluckstein D, Kemper C, et al. A controlled trial of early adjuvant treatment with corticosteroids for Pneumocystis carinii pneumonia in the acquired immunodeficiency syndrome. California Collaborative Treatment Group. N Engl J Med 1990;**323**(21):1451–1457.
[h]Franco-Paredes C, Jacob JT, Stryjewska B, Yoder L. Two Patients with Leprosy and the Sudden Appearance of Inflammation in the Skin and New Sensory Loss. PLoS Negl Trop Dis 2009;**3**(9): e425.
[i]de Gans J, van de Beek D; European Dexamethasone in Adulthood Bacterial Meningitis Study Investigators. Dexamethasone in adults with bacterial meningitis. N Engl J Med 2002;**347**(20):1549–1556.
[j]Powel DR 2nd, Patel S, Franco-Paredes C. Varicella–Zoster Virus vasculopathy: the growing association between herpes zoster and strokes. Am J Med Sci 2015;**350**(3):243–245.

TABLE 16.5 Syndrome of Fever and Anemia and Syndrome of Fever Thrombocytopenia[a,b]

Fever and anemia	Fever and thrombocytopenia
Microorganism directly-related hemolysis	Thrombotic microangiopathy
Malaria	*Escherichia coli Shiga-toxin* (Shiga toxin
Babesiosis	hemolytic uremic syndrome)
Bartonellosis (*Bartonella baciliformis*)	*Shigella dysenteriae* (Shiga toxin
Mycoplasma pneumonia	hemolytic uremic syndrome)
Clostridium perfringens (alpha-toxin-	HIV-associated ADAMTS13 deficiency
lecithinase)	thrombotic microangiopathy (thrombotic
Candida albicans	thrombocytopenic purpura)
Autoimmune hemolytic anemia	Enteropathogens[c]
Mycoplasma pneumoniae (IgM cold-	Shigella may cause thrombocytopenia
antibodies)	with elevated transaminases
Epstein-Barr virus (Infectious	Enteric fever
Mononucleosis)	Rickettsia
Hemophagocytosis	Human granulocytic erlichiosis, Rocky
Infectious-related (ie, viral, TB, or	Mountain spotted fever and human
histoplasmosis)	monocytic anaplasmosis)
Viral	Viral
Red cell aplasia	HIV
Parvovirus B19, Epstein–Barr virus,	Mumps
HTLV-1, HIV, thymomas	Parvovirus B19
Systemic vasculitis	Epstein–Barr virus
(anemia is likely due to chronic	Dengue hemorrhagic fever
inflammation)	Tick-borne Bunyavirus associated-severe
Temporal arteritis	fever and thrombocytopenia syndrome
Adult Onset Still's disease	(similar to Heartland virus)
Rheumatoid arthritis	Hantavirus renal syndrome (even when
Inflammatory	renal failure is absent)
Inflammatory Bowel Disease	Parasitic
Parasitic	*Plasmodium vivax*
Plasmodium vivax	*Plasmodium malariae*
Plasmodium malariae	*P. falciparum*
P. falciparum	Inflammatory
Babesia microti/divergens	Antiphospholipid syndrome
Visceral leishmaniasis *(Leishmania*	Systemic lupus erythematosus
donovani/infantum)	Preeclampsia/HELLP syndrome
	Consumption
	Heparin induced
	Disseminated intravascular coagulation
	Gram-positive or Gram-negative sepsis
	Immune thrombocytopenic purpura
	Destruction
	Mechanical heart valves

[a]*Hemophagocytic syndrome causes pancytopenia. Splenic sequestration may also cause pancytopenia or isolated thrombocytopenia.*
[b]*Evans syndrome is a combination of autoimmune hemolytic anemia and immune-mediated thrombocytopenia.*
[c]*Salmonella* typhi *and S.* Paratyphi A *may also cause leukopenia.*

TABLE 16.6 Leukemoid Reactions Among Immunocompromised Hosts

Leukemoid Reactions > 50,000 cells/mm^3
Disseminated aspergillosis
Disseminated tuberculosis (miliary tuberculosis)
Shigella invasive disease (bacteremia)
Severe and complicated *Clostridium difficile* infection
Drug reaction and eosinophilic systemic syndrome (eosinophilia)
HTLV-1-associated T-cell leukemia lymphoma (lymphocytosis)
Epstein–Barr virus syndromes (infectious mononucleosis and posttransplant
   lymphoproliferative disorder causing lymphocytosis)
Acute retroviral syndrome associated with HIV (lymphocytosis)
Adenovirus type 12 (lymphocytosis)
Pertussis (lymphocytosis)
Drug-induced (corticosteroids)
Hemorrhage (retroperitoneal)

Leukemoid reactions may be present even among immunocompromised hosts, and in fact, these reactions may be more frequently observed among those with some type of immunodeficiency (Table 16.6).

REFERENCES

1. Narins RG, Emmett M. Simple and mixed acid–base disorders: a practical approach. *Medicine* 1980;**59**(3):161–87.
2. Franco-Paredes C, Evans J, Jurado R. Diabetes insipidus due to *Streptococcus pneumoniae* meningitis. *Arch Intern Med* 2001;**161**:1114–5.

Chapter 17

Febrile Syndromes

DIAGNOSTIC APPROACH TO FEBRILE SYNDROMES IN INFECTIOUS DISEASES

Fever is a cardinal clinical sign.[1] Fever results from the elevation of body temperature that exceeds the normal daily variation linked to an increase in the hypothalamic set point and must be distinguished from hyperthermia where an uncontrolled increase in body temperature exceed the body's ability to lose heat (Table 17.1). Some fever patterns may pose clinical significance and may point towards a specific condition (Table 17.2).[1] Night sweats may also be helpful to distinguish infectious causes of fever versus noninfectious causes of fever (Table 17.3). The most likely mechanism of night sweats associated with infectious diseases is an adaptive process by sweat production for the body to reach the nocturnal nadir as part of the circadian rhythm of body temperature.

Syndromic diagnosis of fever in association with other signs or symptoms is a clinically useful strategy in the approach to infectious syndromes. Core concepts in the diagnostic approach of selected febrile syndromes include the following:

- *Mononucleosis and mononucleosis-like illness*: consists of fever, pharyngitis, and lymphadenopathy (Table 17.4)
- *Fever and pancytopenia*: fever in association with anemia, thrombocytopenia, and leukopenia (Table 17.5)
- *Hemophagocytic syndrome*: consists of fever, pancytopenia, elevated transaminases, splenomegaly, hyperferritinemia, and hypertryglicerdemia; and histopathological evidence of hemophagocytosis in the bone marrow, spleen, or lymph nodes without evidence of malignancy (Table 17.6)
- *Fever and arthralgia/arthritis* (Table 17.7)
- *Fever and rash* (Table 17.8)
- *Fever and travel* (see Chapter 14)
- *Prolonged undifferentiated fever (fever of unknown origin)* (Table 17.9)

Core Concepts in Clinical Infectious Diseases (CCCID). http://dx.doi.org/10.1016/B978-0-12-804423-0.00017-2

TABLE 17.1 Differences Between Fever and Hyperthermia

Fever	Elevation of body temperature in adaptation to increase in the hypothalamic set point in response to pyrogenic molecules	Infectious Autoimmune Autoinflammatory Neoplastic
Hyperthermia	Uncontrolled increase in body temperature exceeding the body's ability to lose this heat.	Central nervous system damage (hemorrhage, trauma, status epilepticus) Heat stroke (exertional or nonexertional – anticholinergics, antiparkinsonian drugs, diuretics) Endocrine (thyrotoxicosis, pheochromocytoma **Drug induced** *Serotonin syndrome* (usually normal levels of creatinine phosphokinase – CPK) due to selective serotonin reuptake inhibitors or monoamne oxidase inhibitors, linezolid) *Street drugs* [amphetamines, cocaine, ecstasy (MDMA), salicylates, lithium, anticholinergics] *Neuroleptic malignant syndrome* (dopamine blockers) *Malignant hyperthermia* (inhalational anesthetics, succinylcholine)

TABLE 17.2 Fever Patterns and Associated Clinical Conditions[a]

Fever pattern	Description	Associated diseases
Double quotidian fever	Two paroxysms of fever in 24 h	Visceral leishmaniasis Adult onset Still's disease Miliary tuberculosis Right-sided endocarditis (*Neisseria gonorrhoeae*)
Intermittent fever	Fever that return to normal at least once during most days	Gram-negative bacteremia Intraabdominal abscess Liver abscess Toxic shock syndrome (staphylococci or streptococci) Herpes encephalitis (HSV-1) Acute endocarditis

TABLE 17.2 Fever Patterns and Associated Clinical Conditions (*cont.*)

Fever pattern	Description	Associated diseases
Continuous or sustained fever	Do not vary more than 1°C	Drug fever Central nervous system damage (eg, intraventricular hemorrhage) Kawasaki's disease Macrophage activation syndrome Hemophagocytic syndrome Enteric fever (typhoid fever)
Relapsing fever	Recurrent fever over days or weeks and may have an underlying pattern (intermittent, sustained, remittent)	*Borrelia recurrentis* louse borne *Borrelia. duttoni* tick borne Subacute bacterial endocarditis
Biphasic fever	Two sequential phases	Leptospirosis Dengue hemorrhagic fever Yellow fever West Nile virus Chikungunya Rat-bite fever (*Spirillum minus*) Brucellosis Murine typhus (also Rocky Mountain spotted fever)
Pulse–temperature dissociation (there is no corresponding increase in hear rate to increased temperature ~increase 10 beats per 1°C increase)[b]		*Intracellular pathogens* Tuberculosis (military and acute forms) Brucellosis Enteric fever (typhoid and paratyphoid) *Drug fever*

[a]Cunha BK. *The clinical significance of fever patterns.* Infect Dis Clin North Am 1996;**10**(1):33–42.
[b]Cunha BA, Lortholary O, Cunha CB. *Fever of unknown origin: a clinical approach.* Am J Med 2015;**128**:1138.e1–1138.e15.

TABLE 17.3 Differential Diagnosis of Night Sweats[a]

Febrile	*Infections* (tuberculosis, brucellosis, visceral leishmaniasis, liver abscess, subacute bacterial endocarditis, infectious mononucleosis) *Neoplastic* (Hodgkin's disease, non-Hodgkin's lumphoma) *Systemic inflammatory conditions* (sarcoidosis, IgG-4 related disease, vasculitis) *Drug induced* (niacin, tamoxifen, meperidine, alcohol, antipyretics)
Nonfebrile	*Endocrine* (pheochromocytoma, thyrotoxicosis, carcinoid syndrome, menopause, acromegaly, insulinoma, diabetes mellitus) *Autonomic dysfunction syndromes* (eg, Shy Drager syndrome, familial dysautonomias) *Panic disorder* *Angina*

[a]Franco-Paredes C, Mehrabi D, Calle JC, Jurado RL. *Night sweats revisited.* Infect Dis Clin Practice 2002;**11**(5):291–293.

TABLE 17.4 Etiologies of Infectious Mononucleosis and Mononucleosis-Like Illnesses[a]

Category	Disease	Core concepts
Herpesvirus	Epstein–Barr virus (EBV) Cytomegalovirus (CMV) Epstein–Barr virus (EBV) Human herpes virus-6[b] Herpes simplex virus	More than 90% of cases of IM are caused by EBV
Other viral	HIV	Acute retroviral infection may lead to an IM-like illness characterized by nontender diffuse lymphadenopathy
	Adenovirus (pharyngo-conjunctival fever)	Similar clinical picture as that caused by *Streptococcus pyogenes*
Bacterial	*S. pyogenes* (Group A Streptococci)	Patients present with abrupt onset of pharyngitis, tender and enlarged cervical lymphadenopathy, and fever
Parasitic	*Toxoplasma gondii* (Toxoplasmosis)[c]	A IM-like illness may occur during the acute phase of infection after ingesting of infected undercooked meat with bradyzoites or cysts; or exposure to oocysts in cat feces

[a]*Fever, lymphadenopathy, and pharyngitis. It is important to note that early manifestations of adult onset Still's disease (AOSD) may mimic pharyngitis and fever, but usually is not associated with lymphadenopathy and presents with arthralgias/arthritis.*
[b]*HHV-6 is associated with exanthem subitum and drug reaction eosinophilic systemic syndrome (DRESS)*
[c]*Hurt C, Tammaro D. Diagnostic evaluation of mononucleosis-like illnesses. Am J Med 2007;**120**: 911.e1–911.e8; Lennon P, Crotty M, Fenton JE. Infectious mononucleosis. Brit Med J 2015;**350**:h1825.*

TABLE 17.5 Fever and Pancytopenia Syndromes[a]

Syndrome	Condition	Core concepts/description
Hemophagocytic syndrome	Viral-associated hemo-phagocytic syndrome	Epstein–Barr (other herpes virus) HIV Histoplasmosis Tuberculosis
Malignancy	Acute leukemia (myelo-dysplastic syndromes) Multiple myeloma Infiltration with lymphoma	HTLV-1 associated human T-cell leukemia that is frequently associated with hypercalcemia and pancytopenia
Syndrome of trombothic microangi-opathy	ADAMTS13 deficiency-mediated[b]	Also called thrombotic thrombocytopenic purpura (TTP). It may be associated with pancytopenia

TABLE 17.5 Fever and Pancytopenia Syndromes (*cont.*)

Syndrome	Condition	Core concepts/description
Macrophage activation syndromes	Systemic juvenile idiopathic arthritis (sJIA)[c] Systemic lupus erythematosus Kawasaki disease Periodic fever syndromes	Dysfunctional immune response that is similar to that what is seen in hemophagocytic syndrome (hemophagocytic lymphohistiocytosis)
Bacterial (intracellular) affecting the reticuloendothelial system	Brucellosis (*Brucella melitensis*) Enteric fever (*Salmonella typhi*) Acute disseminated tuberculosis Miliary tuberculosis	Pancyptopenia may occur as a manifestation of fulminant gram-negative or gram-positive associated sepsis
Parasitic	Visceral leishmaniasis	*Leishmania donovani/infantum*
Viral	HIV	Patients with advanced AIDS may have multifactorial pancytopenia (some patients may have concomitant disseminated *Mycobacterium avium-intracellulare*, malnutrition, bone marrow toxicity)
Chronic liver failure	Cirrhosis, portal hypertension, ascites	Pancytopenia may be multifactorial. Patients with spontaneous bacterial peritonitis may not always have fever

[a]*The combination of fever and pancytopenia is associated with infectious causes and noninfectious causes. Of the noninfectious causes, hematologic malignancies are important to consider. Syndromes of macrophage activation or hemophagocytic are also important to consider. Of these two syndromes, the hemophagocytic syndrome maybe associated with an infectious process. Other causes of pancytopenia include megaloblastic anemia, hypersplenism, increased peripheral destruction (splenomegaly), and paroxysmal nocturnal hemoglobinuria*
[b]*George JN, Nester CN. Syndromes of thrombotic microangiopathy. N Engl. J Med 2014;**371**(7): 654–666.*
[c]*This condition is equivalent to adult-onset Still disease (Ravelli A, Davi S, Minoia F, Martini A, Cron RQ. Macrophage activation syndrome. Hematol Oncol Clin N Am 2015;**29**(5):927–941.*

TABLE 17.6 Etiologies and Clinical Features of the Hemophagocytic Syndrome[a]

Category[b]	Disease	Etiologies/description
Infection-associated hemophagocytic syndrome	Virus-associated hemophagocytic syndrome	Herpes viruses (herpes simplex viruses, cytomegalovirus, Epstein–Barr virus, Varicella–Zoster virus, human herpes virus 6, human herpesvirus 8)

(Continued)

TABLE 17.6 Etiologies and Clinical Features of the Hemophagocytic Syndrome (cont.)

Category	Disease	Etiologies/description
	Other infections associated with hemophagocytic syndrome[c]	Other (HIV, adenovirus, parvovirus B19, influenza, hepatitis A) Fungal (histoplasmosis, cryptococcosis, fusariosis, invasive candidiasis) Bacterial and mycobacterial (tuberculosis, BCG infusion bladder carcinoma, *Campylobacter*, legionellosis, typhoid, rickettsial, brucellosis) Parasitic (*L. donovani*, *Plasmodium vivax*, *Plasmodium falciparum*, babesiosis, disseminated strongyloidiasis)
Noninfectious	Primary or genetic	Familial hemophagocytic lymphohistiocytosis Immune deficiency syndromes (Chediak–Higashi syndrome, severe combined immune deficiency, and others)
	Malignancy-associated hemophagyctic lymphohistiocytosis	Lymphoma-associated hemophagocytic lymphohistiocytosis

[a]Hemophagocytic syndrome consists of fever, pancytopenia, elevated transaminases, splenomegaly, hyperferritinemia, and hypertryglicerdemia in association with histopathological evidence of hemophagocytosis in the bone marrow, spleen, or lymph nodes without evidence of malignancy.
[b]Janka GE. Hemophagocytic syndromes. Blood Rev. 2007;**21**:245–253; Rouphael NG, Talati NJ, Vaughan C, Cunningham K, Moreira R, Gould C. Infections associated with haemophagocytic syndrome. Lancet Infect Dis 2007;7:814–822.
[c]Hyperferritinemia usually more than 10,000 occur with the hemophagocytic syndrome and with macrophage activation syndromes.

TABLE 17.7 Fever and Arthralgia/Arthritis

Category	Etiology	Core concepts
Septic arthritis[a]	Gonococcal Nongonococcal (bacterial, parasitic, fungal)	Antimicrobial therapy Requires intravenous antibiotics and drainage (percutaneous or surgical)
Viral arthritis	Parvovirus B19	Acute and symmetric, often metacarphophalangeal and proximal interphalangeal joints of hands. Other areas maybe affected (wrists, kness, ankles, and elbows). If a rash is present, the differential diagnosis is with other viral exanthems and with systemic lupus erythematosus

TABLE 17.7 Fever and Arthralgia/Arthritis (*cont.*)

Category	Etiology	Core concepts
	Rubella	Acute and symmetric, often metacarphophalangeal and proximal interphalangeal joints of hands. Other areas maybe affected (wrists, kness, ankles, and elbows)
	Chikungunya Zika	Patients with Chikungunya may have symptoms for many months (Zika is an emerging arbovirus in the Caribbean and South America)
	HIV and hepatitis C	Reactive arthritis, septic arthritis in HIV-infected individuals. Patients with hepatitis C and cryoglobulinemia may be associated with arthralgias
Reactive arthritis	*Shigella* *Campylobacter jejuni* *Clostridium difficile* *Chlamydia trachomatis*	Usually after 2 weeks of initial episode of gastroenteritis or genital infection. Triggering infection may also be asymptomatic. It may affect large joints (knees, wrist, and elbow) and/or metacarpophalangeal and proximal interphalangeal
	S. pyogenes	Poststreptococcal is frequent and is distinguished from rheumatic fever by acute mono- or oligoarthritis preceded by pharyngitis and history of scarlatiniform rash but absent by the time of arthritis and no other criteria of rheumatic fever
Lyme's arthritis	*Borrelia burgdorferi* *Borrelia garinii* *Borrelia azfelli*	Monoarticular usually affecting large joints (knees, ankle, elbows) and may occur early, but more frequently after untreated chronic disseminated disease with a remissions and relapses
Common variable immune deficiency[b]	History of recurrent sinusitis, bronchiectasis, pneumonia, and hypogammaglobulinemia	Some patients develop a symmetric polyarthritis that often mimics rheumatoid arthritis

(Continued)

TABLE 17.7 Fever and Arthralgia/Arthritis (*cont.*)

Category	Etiology	Core concepts
Gout	Deposition of monosodium urate crystals	Polyarticular with fever and occasionally meeting SIRS criteria. Important to confirm diagnosis and rule out concomitant septic arthritis[c]
Pseudogout	Deposition of calcium pyro-phosphate crystals	
Mycobacterial	Tuberculosis-associated Poncet's disease[d]	Polyarthritis occurring during active pulmonary tuberculosis and affects knees, ankles, and elbows
	Mycobacterium tuberculosis *Mycobacterium kansasii*	Septic arthritis

[a]*See chapter: Osteoarticular Infections, for a detailed discussion of the diagnostic approach of septic arthritis.*
[b]*Abolhassani H, Sagvand BT, Shokuhfar T, Mirminachi B, Rezaei N, Aghamohammadi A. A review of guidelines for management and treatment of common variable immunodeficiency. Expert Rev Clin Immunol 2013;**9**(6):567–575.*
[c]*A patient with gout or pseudogout may have a flare concomitantly with septic arthritis, albeit is a rare association.*
[d]*Franco-Paredes C, Diaz-Borjon A, Barragán L, Senger M, Leonard M. The ever expanding association between tuberculosis and rheumatologic diseases. Am J Med 2006;**119**:470–477.*

TABLE 17.8 Fever and Rash[a]

Category	Etiology	Core concepts[b]
Erythemas confluent with desquamation	Group A Streptococci	Scarlet fever Kawasaki's disease
	Staphylococcus aureus *S. pyogenes*	Toxic shock syndrome (erythema desquamates subsequently)
	Pharyngitis due to *Archanobacterium haemolyticum*	Diffuse erythema, different than scarlet fever
	Drug reactions	Drug reaction eosinophilic systemic syndrome (DRESS)
	Cutaneous lymphoma	Also Sezary syndrome
Petechial	Meningococcemia Rocky Mountain spotted fever	*Neisseria meningitidis* A/C/Y/W-135
	Viral hemorrhagic fevers Gram-negative sepsis	Lassa fever Enterobacteriaceae, *Capnocytophaga canomorsus*, *Streptococcus pneumoniae* or *Haemophilus influenzae* in asplenic
	Acute bacterial endocarditis Enterovirus	*S. aureus*
	Epstein–Barr virus	Mononucleosis or hemophagocytic syndrome

TABLE 17.8 Fever and Rash (*cont.*)

Category	Etiology	Core concepts
Maculopapular	Ehrlichiosis Typhoid fever Viral exanthems Other	Rose spots (seen in the abdominal wall) Rubella, measles, parvovirus B19, cytomegalovirus, HHV-6, enteroviruses Secondary syphilis, Rocky Mountain spotted fever (*Rickettsia rickettsii*) Rat-bite fever (*Streptobacillus monilliformis* or *S. minus*)
Eschar and adenopathy Eschar no adenopathy	Tularemia Anthrax Rickettsialpox Plague Tick-borne spotted rickettsial group	*Francisella tularensis* *Bacillus anthracis* *Rickettsia akari* *Yersinia pestis* *Rickettsia africae* *Rickettsia parkeri*
Nodular lesions	Fungal Mycobacterial Bacterial	(*Candida, Mucor, Fusarium, Sporothrix*, Coccidiodomycosis, Blastomycosis)[c] *Mycobacterium haemophilum, Mycobacterium chelonae, Mycobacterium fortuitum, Mycobacterium marinum* *S. aureus, Nocardia* spp
Vesicular, or vesiculobullous	Chickenpox/Herpes Zoster Rickettsialpox *Vibrio vulnificus*	Varicella–Zoster virus (VZV) – Disseminated *Rickettsia akari* Oyster ingestion in a patient with chronic liver disease or iron excess conditions
Rash with vesicles, pustules, and erosions[d]	Kaposi's varicelliform eruption (eczema herpeticum) Bullous impetigo Folliculitis Cellulitis Chickenpox/Herpes Zoster Eczema vaccinatum Water exposure	Associated with herpes simplex virus (HSV-1) in patients with history of atopic dermatitis. Other associated viruses include HSV-2, vaccinia, cosackievirus A16 *S. aureus* inoculated into areas of dermatitis *S. aureus* Group A Streptococci/Group B Streptococci Varicella–Zoster virus Vaccinia *Erysipelothrix rhusiopathiae* *Aeromonas* spp.

[a]*Schlossberg D. Fever and rash.* Infect Dis Clin North Am *1996;**10**:101–110.*
[b]*It is always crucial identify those patients with fever and rash that may be life-threatening illness.*
[c]*Mackool BT, Governman J, Nazarian RM. Case 14-2012: A 43-year-old woman with fever and generalized rash.* N Engl. J Med *2012;**366**:1825–1834.*
[d]*Cryptococcosis and histoplasmosis produce nodular umbilicated lesions.*

TABLE 17.9 Prolonged Undifferentiated Febrile Syndromes[a,b]

Category	Etiology	Description
Classic fever of unknown (FUO) origin[c]	Malignancy/ neoplastic	Lymphoma, hypernephroma, renal cell carcinoma, leukemias
	Infectious diseases	Miliary tuberculosis, brucellosis, Q fever (*Coxiella burnetti*), enteric fever, intraabdominal/renal abscess, EBV, CMV, bartonellosis (*Bartonella hensellae* endocarditis), extrapulmonary TB
	Rheumatologic/ inflammatory disorders	Adult Still's disease, Giant cell arteritis/temporal arteritis in those more than 50 years, SLE, other systemic vasculitis
	Miscellaneous disorders	Drug fever, cirrhosis, subacute thyroiditis, Crohn's disease
Fever of unknown origin in patients with HIV	Acute HIV	May manifests as a mononucleosis like illness
	Tuberculosis	Primary progressive tuberculosis, active pulmonary, extrapulmonary TB
	Other mycobacterial	Disseminated *Mycobacterium avium-intracellular/M. kansasii*
	Pneumocytis jirovecii (PCP)	Due to its subacute clinical course sometimes falls within FUO
	CMV disease	CMV colitis, esophagitis, gastritis, retinitis, or other
	Disseminated histoplasmosis	May manifest as hemophagocytic syndrome
	Penicillium marneffei	Southeast Asia, Central/South America
	Visceral leishmaniasis Other: *Aspergillus, Bartonella* spp.	In Europe, Africa, associated with intravenous drug use
	Malignancies	Lymphomas, Kaposi's sarcoma (visceral forms without many mucocutaneous manifestations), Multicentric Castleman's disease or primary effusion lymphomas associated with HHSV-8
	Drug fever	Sulfa (colace or cotrimoxazole) Abacavir may produce a hypersensitivity reaction (need to screen with HLA B5701)
	Immune reconstitution syndromes	TB, cryptococcosis, hepatitis, KSHV-MC (Kaposi Sarcoma Herpes virus) inflammatory cytokine syndrome[d]

TABLE 17.9 Prolonged Undifferentiated Febrile Syndromes (*cont.*)

Category	Etiology	Description
Fever of unknown origin in solid organ transplants	Posttransplant lymphoproliferative disorders *Fusarium* *Exophialia* sinusitis *Cryptococcus neoformans* Invasive aspergillosis *P. jirovecii* (PCP) Syndromes of thrombotic microangiopathy[e] Iatrogenic	 ADAMTS13 deficiency-mediated thrombotic microangiopathy (also called thrombotic thrombocytopenic purpura –TTP) West Nile Virus Lymphocytic Choriomeningitis virus
Noninfectious causes of increasingly recognized causes of fever of unknown origin in	IgG-4-related disease with aortitis[f] Giant cell arteritis Adult onset Still's disease	
fever of too many origins[g]	Prolonged intensive care of critically ill patients with a sequence of multi-drug resistant infections (hospital acquired)	These frequent clinical scenarios where using antibiotics in apparently futile situations pose ethical dilemmas

[a]*Brown M. Pyrexia of unknown origin 90 years on: a paradigm of modern clinical medicine.* Postgrad Med J 2015;**0**:1–5.
[b]*Cunha BA, Lortholary O, Cunha CB. Fever of unknown origin: a clinical approach.* Am J Med 2015;**128**:1138.e1–1138.e15.
[c]*Petersdorf and Beeson developed criteria for prolonged fevers: fever greater than 38.3°C for more than 3 weeks that remains undiagnosed after a inpatient hospital workup. The 3-week mark referred to the fact that some viral infections, in particular Epstein–Barr virus or CMV may completely defervesce within a period of 1–3 weeks.*
[d]*Polizzotto MN, Uldrick TS, hu D, Yarchoan R. Clinical manifestations of Kaposi sarcoma herpesvirus lytic activation: multicentric Castleman disease (KSHV-MCD) and the KSHV inflammatory cytokine syndrome.* Front Microbiol 2012;**3**(73):1–9.
[e]*There are inherited and acquired thrombotic microangiopathy syndromes (George JN, Nester CN. Syndromes of thrombotic microangiopathy. N Engl. J Med 2014;**371**(7):654–666.).*
[f]*Kanisawa T, Zen Y, Pillai S, Stone JH. IgG4-related disease.* Lancet 2015;**385**(9976):1460–1471.
[g]*Horowitz HW. Fever of unknown origin or fever of too many origins?* N Engl. J Med 2013;**368**(3):197–199.

REFERENCE

1. Mackowiak PA, Bartlett JG, Borden EC, Goldblum SE, Hasday JD, Munford RS, et al. Concepts of fever: recent advances and lingering dogma. Clin Infect Dis 1997;25:119–38.

Subject Index

A

ABPA. *See* Allergic bronchopulmonary aspergillosis (ABPA)
Abscesses, 9, 25, 85
  brain, 25
  formation, 1
  intraabdominal, 9
  liver, 85
  pituitary, 205
Acanthamoeba, 33
Acetaminophen, 86, 114
Acid–base disorders, 201
  and infectious diseases, 201
Acute generalized exanthematous pustulosis (AGEP), 114
Acute phase reactants, 6
Adrenal glands, 206, 207
Adrenal hemorrhage, 207
Adult-onset Still's disease (AOSD), 127
African trypanosomiasis, 177
AGEP. *See* Acute generalized exanthematous pustulosis (AGEP)
Allergic bronchopulmonary aspergillosis (ABPA), 59
Amazonian river, 1
Amyloidosis, 149
  organ-specific, 149
    cardiac amyloidosis, 149
    hepatic amyloidosis, 149
    nephritic, 149
Anemia, 158, 189, 207, 209, 211
Angioedema, 114, 124, 180, 191, 193
  selected causes of, 124
Angiotensin-converting-enzyme inhibitors, 114
Animal bites, infections associated with, 115
Animal exposure, infections associated with, 115
Ankylosing spondylitis, 53
Anogenital warts/carcinomas differential diagnosis, 102
Anogenital warts/carcinomas, clinical spectrum, 102
Antibody deficiency, 187
  etiology and differential diagnosis of immunodeficiencies, 189

Anticytokine antibodies, 191
  category and diseases/syndromes, 191
  clinical spectrum of immunodeficiencies, 191
Antifactor H autoantibodies, 191
Anti-GM-CSF autoantibodies, 59
Antigranulocyte-macrophage colonystimulating factor (anti-GM-CSF), 56, 58
Anti-IL-17 autoantibodies, 191
Antimicrobial interventions, 1
Antimicrobial susceptibility, 51
Antiretroviral drugs, 79
AOSD. *See* Adult-onset Still's disease (AOSD)
Apoptosis, 51
Archanobacterium haemolyticum, 45
Arthralgia, 127, 142, 183, 216
Arthritis, 12, 71, 118, 127, 130, 143, 189
Ascending paralysis, differential diagnosis of, 27
Aspergillus fumigatus, 53
Aspergillus nidulans, 191
Autoantibodies, 118, 188
  to C1 inhibitor, 191
Autoimmunity, 157
Autoinflammation, 157

B

Babesiosis, 1
Bacteremia, 1, 7, 9, 63
  caused by *S. aureus*, 11
Bacteria community-associated *methicillin* resistant *Staphylococcus aureus*, 53
Bacterial endocarditis, 9
Bacterial meningitis, 23, 205
  acute, 20
Bacterial rhinosinusitis, complications of, 45
Batson's venous plexus, 137
B-cell lymphoproliferative disorders, 187
BCG vaccination, 191
Beta-lactam drugs, 114
Bisphosphonate-related osteonecrosis of the jaw (BRONJ), 138
Bisphosphonates, 138

Printed in the United States
By Bookmasters